The A to Z of Loss:
The handbook for healthcare

Elizabeth Bell
Psychologist

Foreword by
Emma Storr

Radcliffe Publishing
Oxford • Seattle

10-05

Radcliffe Publishing Ltd
18 Marcham Road
Abingdon
Oxon OX14 1AA
United Kingdom

www.radcliffe-oxford.com
Electronic catalogue and worldwide online ordering facility.

British Library Cataloguing in Publication Data

A catalogue record for this book is available from the British Library.

ISBN 1 85775 653 3

Typeset by Aarontype Ltd, Easton, Bristol
Printed and bound by TJ International Ltd, Padstow, Cornwall

To Paul, Rosemary and Dr Kathryn Jennings

There are no pockets in shrouds

Contents

Foreword

The A to Z of Loss should be on every healthcare professional's shelf. At the heart of the book is a concern to understand the experience of 'loss' amongst our clients and patients. We will rarely be able to change the circumstances that have led to this experience but, as professionals involved in their care, we will be more effective and helpful to them if we can appreciate the many 'losses' that make up everyday life.

The chapters in this book are organised on an alphabetical theme (A is for Anxiety, B is for Baby, etc) and each of the 26 scenarios provides a story about an individual and their particular experience. We encounter the familiar losses of bereavement and illness, but also those of a more subtle nature, such as the loss of dignity or power. At the end of each narrative, a short discussion of the psychological points is followed by a series of challenging questions that encourage personal and professional development. Answering these questions requires a deep level of analysis and thinking, as well as a willingness to confront our own prejudices and assumptions. It will be salutary for anyone involved in healthcare to consider these points, as well as using them when teaching students.

I can imagine dipping in and out of this book and using the different stories to teach and engage students in any of the caring professions. Healthcare education now includes training in communication skills and this is even more essential as we deal with an increasingly well-informed and sophisticated public. As a handbook to aid in this process, *The A to Z of Loss* provides invaluable advice, which is both accessible and sensible.

Dr Emma Storr
General Practitioner
Senior Teaching Fellow
Academic Unit of Primary Care
University of Leeds
December 2004

About the author

Elizabeth Bell is a psychologist and author who taught the psychology of healthcare at Leeds University for nine years. She graduated from University College London, took a postgraduate certificate of education (PGCE) from Oxford University and completed her training as an educational psychologist with an MSc from Manchester University in the 1980s. She enjoys playing the piano and has made several CDs for the charity The Medical Foundation for the Care of the Victims of Torture.

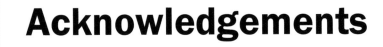

Acknowledgements

I would like to thank the people (names have been changed to preserve anonymity) who contributed their accounts to these scenarios. It is recognised that many changes have taken place within the NHS towards a greater understanding of individual needs. However the need for *sensitivity* remains and perhaps this book can serve as a reminder, in an increasingly hectic world, that no time is ever wasted in the establishment of rapport.

I would also like to thank Gillian Nineham (Editorial Director) and the team at Radcliffe Publishing, Sarah Hodgson (Alzheimer's Society), Joseph Peate (author's photograph and technological support), EA Haighton, Gill Scott, Susannah Marshall (cartoonist), Catherine Torjussen, Padraic Monaghan, Sue Campbell, Stuart Davies and Yelena Konyukh.

Introduction

Illness is the night-side of life, a more onerous citizenship. Everyone who is born holds dual citizenship, in the kingdom of the well and in the kingdom of the sick. Although we all prefer to use only the good passport, sooner or later each of us is obliged, at least for a spell, to identify ourselves as citizens of that other place.[1]

(Excerpt from *Illness as Metaphor* by Susan Sontag. Copyright © 1977, 1978 by Susan Sontag. Reprinted by permission of Farrar, Straus and Giroux, LLC.)

To 'identify ourselves as citizens of that other place' means to suffer the loss of well-being. From minor ailments, such as the common cold, to admission to an intensive care unit (ICU), we sense the loss of our selves as fully functioning people. The threat to our identity will vary: a cold may make us feel slightly under the weather, whereas to recover consciousness after a road traffic accident (RTA) in an ICU is a more threatening experience. Even after a sense of relief, having survived an admission to an ICU, our minds may be full of questions (What's happened to me? Where am I? Am I going to die?) that we may not be able to articulate.

We will also vary, as individuals, in the degree to which we are vulnerable to loss at any particular time. People who have suffered many losses in life may be more vulnerable; people who are sensitive may feel things deeply; people who are less sensitive, and possibly fortunate as well, may not be able to appreciate the pain that loss and the ensuing grief incurs. But as healthcare professionals, we need to be able to humanise what may be the psychologically damaging effects of the hi-tech equipment (and thinking?) in medicine today. We also need to be able to access empathetic support for what may seem to us to be very minor problems. And, to sustain the ability to work across the range of experiences of loss, we do, of course, need to look after ourselves.

Loss, or rather the *sense of loss*, has to be one of the hardest psychological problems that faces human beings. Why? I think that we can explore this question at three levels:

- the psychological
- the sociological
- the political.

Psychologically, we are unique as a species in spending so much time in a position of dependency as we mature. We are therefore relying on the quality of the attachments that we make in childhood to secure our emotional futures as adults. Loss of 'quality care' in childhood may leave us vulnerable to relationship breakdowns in adult life. The word 'attachment' suggests belonging and even possession, and yet, as adults, if we operate on the basis of trying to possess the people we love, relationships may be strangled. We all need a sense of belonging, but if we put all our emotional eggs in one basket, we are usually forced to manipulate that relationship; the strain of too many demands on it can lead to its eventual breakdown. Bowlby[2] used the term 'bonding' and he highlighted the damage to adult relationships if children did not receive adequate parental care. Attachment, belonging, possessing, bonding – the strength of these terms reflects the need we have to relate, to connect with one another. We live in a society in the twenty-first century which seems obsessed with 'relationships', but usually in the sense of an intense 'one-on-one' bias. At what emotional risk (of the pain of loss) do we place ourselves, if we believe that the answer to our needs can only be found in and through somebody else? And what sort of society do we create if we think that whoever we are with is not quite enough, and that there is always AN Other, just around the next corner? And what is the cost to health services of the stresses from the fall-out from relationship breakdown?

Sociologically, in the last 50 or so years, we have changed from a society in which the family stayed together to one that is likely to contain a mixture of step parents and step children. For example, in 1995, the UK had the second highest divorce rate in the EU (after Belgium) and, in 1999, there was one divorce for every two marriages.[3] These people have experienced relationship breakdown and their 'baggage' is likely to include emotional debris from the past (particularly the emotions associated with loss and the grieving of that loss: sadness, guilt, anger, regret, to name but some). It was interesting to observe the nationwide grief for the death of Princess Diana in August 1997. How strange it was to see people crying in public for somebody that they had never known. Could it be that the death of the celebrity princess permitted people to grieve publicly; a grief, the source of which was the nation's identification with Diana's difficult life, in terms of relationships; a grief that is still reluctantly expressed in a country of the 'stiff upper lip'? And so there is a sense in which we inhabit a country of contradictions: relationships are sold to us through the media while relationship breakdowns are the content of soap operas. We might be forgiven for being confused: it is almost the norm for breakdowns to occur and yet somewhere in our consciousness there may be the memory of times when families stayed together.

Politically, as global capitalism accelerates, we are insidiously persuaded that 'having' (more and more material possessions) takes precedence over 'being' (a person with sufficient but not excessive access to global resources). Further, 'having' requires a huge commitment to being busy ('doing') which can lead to people suffering the sense of loss of time, the loss of time to enjoy the money which they have earned. It is a vicious circle. All of us are engaged, to a greater or lesser degree, in balancing these three processes or paths:

- *being*
- *having*
- *doing*.

It is arguable that too much investment in *'doing and having'* is unhealthy. First of all, the pressures create stressful lifestyles. 'Stress-related conditions count for more than half of all disability' in northern European countries.[4]

Second, to identify ourselves with what we do (e.g. our jobs) and what we own (e.g. clothes, cars, houses; if not an attempt at possession of the people in our lives) makes us vulnerable to the loss of these things. In a society, in a world, which increasingly sells the message that to be successful means to be happy and that to be identified as a success means to be a very-busy-person-with-a-lot-of-stuff, we are increasingly vulnerable to the fear of being identified as 'losers'. 'Losers': the word says it all. The image it conveys is of somebody who has failed, who has lost their way in the aspirational climb and who, in some way, suffers the grief from that loss.

However, in the final analysis, we are who we are. We are the bodies we 'inhabit', not forgetting our minds which are full of the best interpretations that we can make of the increasingly complex world around us. It goes without saying, that it is our *being* which keeps us alive, if it can be put like that! It is our loss of the sense of well-being that makes us seek help, from a telephone call to NHS Direct, a trip to the pharmacy, a visit to a walk-in centre, an appointment in primary care or with a complementary therapist, or an admission to hospital.

We are conditioned, in the West, to seek help. We are used to perceiving ourselves as patients and the medical profession as experts (even though many of us may access the internet too), experts who find out what is wrong with us and then provide a solution to the problem, often highly interventionist. This way of thinking may be apt for some purely physical problems, but if we aspire to holistic medicine then it is the needs of the whole person which must be taken into account. Traditional medicine 'pathologises' suffering by diagnosing and labelling conditions. We need to think beyond the 'appendix in bed three' to the whole person (including the mind). And, in the case of people whose minds would seem to be the primary source of their suffering, we need to change our language. Perhaps instead of the term 'mental', which is stigmatising, we can think of this suffering as 'intangible'. There is a long way to go, educating people away from Cartesian thinking. JK Rowling, perhaps unwittingly, has made this journey longer in her popular Harry Potter books.

> *"He is mental", Fred said.* (Fred to George, speaking about Harry)[5]
> *"You're mental", said George.* (George to Harry)[5]
> *"You're both mental."* (Ron Weasley to Sirius Black and Professor Lupin)[6]

Further, the language of medicine is a language of power. How many people have sufficient knowledge of Latin, let alone science, to understand the pronouncements of some diagnoses, for example *Pityriasis rosea* (*see* page 32)? It is not just a power over words, it is a power over our ability to think clearly for ourselves about what is wrong with us. When Wittgenstein spoke of philosophy being the battle against the bewitchment of our intelligence by means of language, he was offering a solution to this problem.

We need to recall the power of the mind to affect clinical outcomes. Perhaps if we engage with patients' minds, we can engage as true partners in the healing processes which lie at the heart of all recovery. Was it not Voltaire who said that the art of medicine lies in keeping the patient amused while Nature takes its course?

We need to think more clearly about the training (and education) of doctors and nurses. It would seem to be in something of a muddle. Medical students have communication skills workshops squeezed into a tight curriculum, while nursing students attend academically aspirational courses when many of them want to be out in hospitals and surgeries getting on with the job of care. Schools of healthcare studies suffer from being under three masters:

- universities (which aim to maintain academic standards)
- NHS trusts (which want people who can *do* the job of nursing)
- the Nursing and Midwifery Council (a conservative body with considerable control over the curriculum).

The muddle is not just confined to the training of healthcare professionals. Because we are conditioned to be consumers of the health services, we (inadvertently?) contribute to their misuse. For example, *Case Notes* on Radio Four in 2004 reported that in one A&E department in London, 3500 people a day go for help, 700 of whom are at an inappropriate point of access. It is essential that we sort out the confusion so that resources are not wasted. The World Health Organization is warning us now about the predicted increase in 'mental' health problems, for example:

'450 million people worldwide currently suffer from such conditions, placing mental disorders among the leading causes of ill health … depressive disorders, the fourth leading cause of disease and disability, are expected to rank second by 2020 … some 33.4 million people in the WHO European region suffer from major depression in any given year … '.[4]

We also need to recognise the stress that the medical profession has undergone, due to the fall-out from the Thatcherite years (1979–1997). We need to regain respect, as a nation, for the number of hours spent by hardworking individuals in the cause of keeping us alive and healthy. The following quotation taken from the *British Medical Journal* on 17 April 2004, from Pippa Keech, a GP in Southampton, gives us cause both to hope and to despair, hope in that she has 'come out' and admitted such a thing, despair that it took so long:

> 'It has taken me ten years of general practice to see patients as people and not as diseases.'[7]

In this handbook, I am offering the reader a *psychological* analysis of loss, through the presentation of a series of clinical scenarios. Reflective questions for personal and professional development follow each analysis. Each scenario is designed to hold 'hidden losses'. Anybody who is ill has not just lost their immediate well-being. They may be holding a history of loss. If the golden rule is: do unto others as you would be done by, the platinum rule is: do unto others as they would have you do unto them. The rationale therefore is for greater *sensitivity* between patient and professional.

On a more positive note, it is worth remembering that 'loss' is an essential part of life anyway, in the sense that to move forward on the journey is to 'lose' the place from which you have come. Life is about change, and change is a kaleidoscope of loss and gain. The difficulty lies, I believe, in that we are all (patients, carers, professionals) much more comfortable with tangible losses than 'intangibles'. We can justifiably grieve over the loss of a child, but it is not as acceptable perhaps to have a sense of grief over a loss of dignity, status, privacy or opportunity. Many losses we might not even be able to articulate ourselves; there may be shadows from long ago, and even a sense of failure that we still carry such 'baggage'.

In writing for 'healthcare professionals', it is recognised that readers will be coming from a wide range of backgrounds. The format of this book – scenario, analysis-of-the-scenario, questions for professional development – is designed to enable the reader (with or without formal psychological training) to *think* like a psychologist. The word 'therapy' derives from 'attending'. We need to listen, not just with our ears, but with our eyes, our minds, our whole being.

Now myrth now sorrow
Now dolour then gladnesse
Now better now worse
Now plesure then payne
Now to want then to have
Now love then disdeyne
Now ebbe now flowe
Now corrupte now pure
Now hote now colde
Now drought now rayne

13th century lyric

Author's note: If there is any concern, while reading this book, that it is the author's intent to blame individual healthcare professionals, that would be a misconstruction. If anything is to 'blame', it is the failure of systems, in general, to become the gestalts they might be. Gestalt psychology states that the whole is greater than the sum of the parts. Sadly, in institutions it is all too often the case that not only is the sum of the parts greater than the whole, but some of the parts are greater than the sum.

References

1 Sontag S (1978) *Illness as Metaphor*. Vintage, London.

2 Bowlby J (1953) *Child Care and the Growth of Love*. Pelican, London.

3 www.about.com The Office for National Statistics. 1 August, 2004.

4 WHO (2003) *Mental health in the WHO European Region*. Fact sheet EURO/03/03. World Health Organization, Geneva.

5 Rowling JK (2000) *Harry Potter and the Goblet of Fire*. Bloomsbury, London, p. 635.

6 Rowling JK (1999) *Harry Potter and the Prisoner of Azkaban*. Bloomsbury, London. p. 256.

7 Keech P (2004) Telling it how it is. *BMJ*. **328**: 918.

A is for Anxiety

'They took him down at ten o'clock in the morning. I was only allowed to go with him as far as the lift. He'd been in so much pain with his knees and we were both grateful that his name had finally got to the top of the waiting list for knee replacement surgery. The orthopaedic surgeon had not bothered with me when we went to see him. My husband and he just joked about what playing rugby in your youth can do to your joints.

I was told to go home and wait and that he would be back from the operating theatre and fully conscious by the early afternoon. I could not concentrate on anything. I did not dare go into the garden because I was scared I would miss the phone call from the hospital and also because Bill had been working so hard out there, it would only remind me of him. I kept picturing him unconscious, powerless and defenceless. I'd only ever seen surgery on television. I remembered seeing the surgeon wielding a saw over the patient's leg. I'd also been on the internet and found out how dangerous just having an anaesthetic is. I thought about Bill not admitting to the hospital that he had had a bit of a chest infection the previous week.

I wandered around the house. There were so many photographs of our family together. I had not been able to get hold of our daughter, to tell her about dad's operation. She was up the Amazon, as far as we knew. We had lost our only son when he was just a baby. Nobody at the hospital had been able to tell us exactly what happened. He had just been taken in with fits and then died, alone, in the night on the children's ward.

When I had not heard from the hospital by three o'clock, I had to ring them. They sounded positive but said that he had not yet come back from theatre. I wanted to know why but they sounded really busy. I decided to drive over. I did not have the right change for the Pay and Display car park. By the time I got to the ward, I was beginning to panic. They said that there had been a 'slight problem' and so it was best to get a cup of tea and wait. The last thing I needed was to be sitting in a crowded cafeteria with a cup of bright-orange tea. But I'd not eaten anything since the night before and I was beginning to feel light-headed. After a depressing half-hour surrounded by a mixture of patients, outpatients, relatives and the occasional doctor (and they did all look about 16 years old), I went back to the ward. There was still no information. I could not take any more *uncertainty*. I needed some facts, even if they were facts that nobody wants to hear. The nurse who seemed to be in charge, well, she had Staff Nurse written on her badge and so I guessed that she was in charge of the rest of the staff, was very pleasant but she could not tell me what was happening. I asked if I could go down to the operating theatre and find out for myself. She suggested that I could sit in her office. I was relieved to be in a private area because I was near to tears. It was such a shock when a nurse in a different uniform came in and sat down beside me and just quietly handed me a box of tissues. It turned out that she was not a fully trained nurse at all but she understood just how terrible the *uncertainty* was. The next half-hour seemed to pass really quickly and suddenly I was called out of the office and Bill was returning on the trolley.

Several weeks later, we found out that the surgeon had used the wrong 'cement' on his new joint and had had to break and re-set the leg. That was why he had been so long in the operating theatre. Neighbours said that we should have complained formally to the hospital. But we were just so grateful to have come through safely. I say 'we' but really it is Bill that has come through. I have had to have a course of sleeping tablets from my GP. I admitted that I had always had problems with my nerves and she did offer me counselling but there was a waiting list. I don't know why, but every night I have nightmares about being unable to find my family down the long winding corridors of a hospital, which is only partially constructed, some-where in South America.'

Worry is the dark room where negatives are developed.

Psychological issues

The first thing that we notice is the use of 'us' and 'them' language. She also uses the term 'allowed' as if she is a child.

Then we get the impression of gratitude for rising up the waiting list, followed by uneasiness in the presence of the surgeon who did not include the wife in the discussion.

Now we read that she is 'sent home' and, with insufficient distractions or support, her mind wanders towards the negative end of the spectrum. We also witness the power of television and the internet in 'informing' this woman about what may be happening to her husband.

Having tried being outside, leaving the constrictions, physically and psychologically, of the four walls, she returns to the house. But now photo-graphs attract her attention and she experiences feelings of isolation relating to her inaccessible daughter and memories of the mysterious death of her only son in a hospital many years ago.

Trying not to be a bother to the busy-sounding staff, she sets off for the hospital in person only to experience the unnecessary hassle of parking fees. From now on, we can observe that her perceptions are increasingly negative until she is offered a private place and, by chance, a sympathetic and supportive member of staff.

The label 'Staff Nurse' is misleading. It gives her the impression that the nurse is probably in a managerial role over other staff, and so raises her expectations – which are then disappointed.

The use of the telephone for exchanging clinical information is limited. There is no 'body language' available to convey the wider aspects of the message. Voice is the only thing that can be manipulated. She perceives this to be 'busy-sounding'.

Finding out why things had been so *uncertain* weeks after the event, they decide not to take any action, even though she is suffering the aftermath of the strain and having to purchase prescription drugs.

Personal and professional development

1 How would you limit the effects of 'us' and 'them' thinking in healthcare?
2 Imagine you were the nurse-in-charge of that ward. What would you have done differently?
3 Reflect on your experience of hospital care, either as a patient or as a close friend or relative.
4 She finds the necessary emotional support late in the day, by chance and from somebody who is not fully trained. She and her husband are still grateful, weeks later, for surviving the experience. What does this say about expectations and the rhetoric about 'patients as partners'?
5 Reflect on the sexism and ageism ... and suggest ways of mitigating the effects of these in a clinical setting.
6 Reflect on the effect of the internet as a source of medical information (quality and quantity) disempowering the medical profession.
7 What are the training implications for surgeons in this example?
8 Examine the literature for the research on stress, specifically, the idea of 'daily hassles', and link this with the necessity or otherwise of car-parking fees at hospitals.
9 Think of other situations where *uncertainty* is the key factor, for example waiting for the news of a fire disaster, air crash, earthquake or terrorist attack. What do relatives and friends need at this time?

10 Critically evaluate the offer of counselling (in general and in this example), particularly when there is a waiting list.

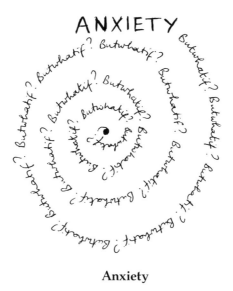

Anxiety

Useful tip
Smile when answering the telephone … you will sound warmer and more helpful.

B is for Baby

'I'd been desperate to conceive another child. We had a son and we wanted a sibling for him and we were also down for adoption. I come from a big family and my husband's very easy-going, so I'd always pictured a big noisy chaotic family with my husband calm and in control. After six years of trying, we conceived. I was convinced it would be another boy. They recommended amniocentesis because I was 40 years old by then, but we would never have aborted a child. The pregnancy went well and I had my date for a Caesarean (Tom had had to be delivered by section and they didn't want to take any risks) but a week before, my waters broke at 0730. Neighbours took Tom to school and Paul drove me to the hospital. The labour pains were excruciating but wonderful because I was giving birth to new life. But they still decided to give me a 'spinal' and the next minute my legs collapsed and off we went to theatre. Fully conscious, all I could feel was a tugging sensation in my abdomen. Then suddenly I was handed a beautiful little girl. In the recovery room, she was put to my breast and although she snuffled a bit, she drank a little milk. She was taken for her Apgar score, got 9, and Paul left me to go and get Tom from school. All four of us sat on the bed together, a perfect little family. I was crying and laughing at the same time. Paul took Tom to get a snack from the hospital cafeteria and I just stared at the miracle, the little scrap of baby at my side. Suddenly the door flew open and a woman said "Your baby looks a bit blue. Was your first child floppy like this at birth? We're taking her to Special Care". And with that, she picked up my baby and left the room. What was going on? Who was she?

That was how we learnt that we had a baby with Down's syndrome. The woman had been a midwife. Paul returned with Tom. Both looked pale. The next minute we were told that Leila had heart problems and would need surgery, and that we would have to go by ambulance to the city hospital. But that turned out to be 'not yet'. It was just chaos. I was so angry that I ran down to Special Care. The nurses were fantastic. They hugged me and held my hand. I wanted to feed Leila but she was on special monitoring for fluids because of her heart. One of the nurses said she'd let me feed her if we hid behind a curtain. Having my baby to my breast and feeding her was what we both needed, but then we heard the doctor coming and had to stop quickly. I could not believe what was happening. One minute we were the perfect family and the next we were fighting for our baby's life. On the third day, I cracked. I could not stop crying. Paul was taking it very differently. He looked like he had been punched in the stomach. A different midwife sat with me and I cried and cried until there were no more tears left. The doctor who had done the Apgar test came in. He apologised for not noticing that Leila had Down's syndrome. He was very young, looked newly qualified and could not have been more sensitive.

Two months later we went with Leila in her incubator in an ambulance to the city for heart surgery. I felt every bump in the road. The heart surgeon was a woman, which made me feel better somehow, even if she did talk about my baby as a 'case' to be 'monitored'. By this time, Paul and I had disregarded the Down's syndrome. We just wanted her to live. She did, covered in tubes and wires.

It's now two years on. We didn't bother to adopt, even though we were accepted. I'm learning sign language. Tom loves his little sister. Paul and I are closer than ever, even though we did grieve so very differently. How can I protect my daughter from people taking advantage of her? What about when we die? We went to a solicitor to make a will and to give custody of Leila to Tom when he is 18 years old. The solicitor started to write that my daughter 'suffers' from Down's syndrome. I would not let him say that. What do we know about her suffering or otherwise? I've learnt a lot in the last few years. Down's children aren't happy all the time either!'

Psychological issues

The key issue here is how *not* to give bad news. Not only is the mother on her own when she is panicked that there is something wrong, but the person giving the news does not introduce herself or her clinical role. The word 'floppy' is also alarming because the link between 'floppiness' and Down's syndrome would probably be made very quickly in a new mother's mind. Similarly, 'your baby looks a bit blue' would cue any parent into fear for the imminent survival or otherwise of their newborn. On the other hand, the clinician has to act quickly in the presence of an emergency case.

Before the conception and delivery, there is also the psychological 'build-up' of yearning for another child. Six years, or six-times-twelve disappointments are not to be taken lightly, particularly for a woman in her 30s. We might question the ostensible reason for wanting another baby as a 'sibling for our son'. There is so much social expectation for couples to have one baby and, per-haps even more so, to have two. We could speculate that this woman is wanting to re-create the big family from whence she came, and why not? We could argue that it is every woman's right to have as many children as she can conceive. But should we not also reflect on the responsibilities of parenthood?

The communication about the heart operation is given at the wrong time, causing more stress, which comes out as anger in the mother. Then we have the collusive breast-feeding incident in Special Care. Meanwhile it is emerging that the mother and her husband, Paul, are very different personalities when it comes to grieving. She is expressive, he is quiet and we are left to imagine what Tom their son is making of all of this. Does he know that this baby was conceived partly for him?

There are also two good incidents. Firstly, there is the second midwife who stays with the mother as she cries, and secondly, the young doctor who bravely apologises for the misleading Apgar score.

Finally, we get a picture of an intact family preparing for an unknown future. The mother is coming across stereotypes about disabled children and taking them head on.

This example is included because the reader might expect to read about the loss of a baby through childbirth, accident or illness but here we have the 'loss of the perfect baby'. We have the shock of a complete shift in expectations.

Personal and professional development

1 Research the literature on Down's syndrome, particularly the impact on the whole family.
2 How do you think the news should have been given to this family?
3 What do you make of the collusive breast-feeding incident?
4 Imagine yourself in the shoes of the mother when she is at home alone for the first time with Leila. How would you help her if you were her health visitor?
5 Many people have a second child as a sibling for the first. What do you think about this?
6 Speculate on the short, medium and long term effects for Tom of having a sister with Down's syndrome.
7 Reflect on the attitudes of society to children with disabilities.
8 Think of different disabilities – autism, spina bifida, cerebral palsy, etc. Do you find it easier/harder to cope with some than others?
9 How would you rate the validity of these reasons for having children?
   - Everyone else has them, so it must be the right thing to do.
   - If I never had children, I might regret it later.
   - My mum would never forgive me if I did not give her grandchildren.

- I've always loved cuddling babies.
- I'm sure my partner will stay with me if I get pregnant.
- An only child is a lonely child, so we'd better have another one.
- If you have three, the middle one gets left out.

(You might like to add your own reasons and reflect on them.)

10 Recall the language of disability – 'special needs', 'learning disabilities'. What do you think of such labels?

Useful tip

Always introduce yourself and your role even if you are wearing a badge.

C is for Child

'I started having these headaches. I put them down to stress. I was having to bring my daughter up on my own and the only job I could get was working for a cosmetics company selling their new range of products. I'd never dared ring in sick just for headaches so I'd told them it was migraines. That way, I could always get out when I needed to. The last thing your boss wants is you being sick all over your business suit. I was out on the road a lot, driving up and down motorways, stuck in traffic jams and worrying about Sara settling in at her new school. She had had to join the secondary school in Year Ten and she had always found it hard to make friends because she was shy. Sometimes she didn't seem like my daughter at all, because I am really outgoing and she is quiet.

Things came to a head one weekend when I was at a sales conference and the presenter was delivering statistics. *30 000 miles of lipstick*, he said, were sold every year across the world. I had just seen a programme the night before about millions of starving children. I thought back to Sara when she was a child and how great she had been and how difficult she was becoming as a teenager. I ran out of the hotel, got in the car, and drove home breaking all the speed limits. Sara was out, a scrawled message on the kitchen table, an empty bottle of vodka by the breadbin.

I drank myself to sleep that night. Sara didn't come home until Sunday afternoon. She refused to speak to me, slammed her bedroom door and didn't come out until I persuaded her to have some tea. We sat in silence. These moods had been going on for months, I realised. I was frightened of the mixed feelings I had for her as she sat there:

- envy of her youthful looks
- anger at the power she had over me by not speaking
- loss of the child she had once been
- guilt that I could not protect her.

On the Monday, she refused to go to school, saying that everybody said she was fat. My boss rang me to sack me and the company car had been scratched in the night. I rang the surgery to get an appointment but they could not fit me in until Thursday. I rang NHS Direct; my head was killing me by now, and

a computer voice cut in. I slammed down the phone. I took some Anadin©
and left the house. I began to feel sick as I walked into town. My eyes were
blurred and I could not tell if it was because I was so near to tears or
something wrong with my head. It was then that I saw the sign for the
Alternative Medical Centre. The receptionist was so friendly and the waiting
area so calm and peaceful, I was happy to sit and wait for a consultation.

After a short wait, the therapist came to collect me. She was warm and
kind, with a big smile and such a good listener. I could not stop crying. I told
her everything: about how I'd been suddenly left by my partner, about Sara's
loss of weight, my loss of job, and even about the way I was beginning to
need to have a bit of a drink to help me get to sleep. She never looked as if
she was judging me at all, even though I was really trying to tell her that Sara
was anorexic and I'm virtually an alcoholic. I never got round to mentioning
the real reason for my visit: the headaches.

After a very long consultation, we got to talking about how I was going
through a 'mid-life crisis', she said, just at the time when my daughter's
hormones were probably clashing with mine. Well, I was 45 years old and
Sara was 14 years old. She told me all about how she had suffered just the
same sort of thing as I was going through. She said that I would need a series
of consultations to 'work through' all my feelings. I never bothered to ask
about her qualifications or the cost at the beginning of the appointment. I was
just so grateful to be able to find somebody who would listen to me.

I left the Alternative Medical Centre, feeling just like my old self. I was
confident. I would get another job easily. My headache had gone. Sara and I
would work things out together, just like we always had. She was not really
anorexic, she was just a typical self-conscious teenager. And I was not a
heavy drinker. But when I got home, Sara was still locked in her bedroom.
Her school bag was hanging on the outside of the door, a bottle of slimming
tablets, *Fatbusters*, sticking out of one of the pockets. I went down into the
lounge and pulled out the old photograph album and cried. She had been such
a lovely kid. Where had the child I once knew gone to?'

Psychological issues

We usually think of the loss of a child as the loss-through-death. This scenario
shows a subtler loss, that of a mother who is struggling with the *loss-of-the-
child-within-the-teenager*. She is also finding it hard to relate to such a close
blood relative who is emerging as somebody with a very different
personality. (Why should we expect relatives to be similar to ourselves?)

The mother is struggling financially, and with a conflict between her deeper
values and her means of earning a living. She is also suffering from the

intensity of a mother/daughter lone-parent relationship at a time when hormones are playing a powerful part in both their lives. She is lying about her headaches at work. By naming them 'migraines', she is using the power of a medical label to gain herself some approved reasons for not going into work. (How many millions of working days are lost per annum in Britain due to stress-related illness? In *Burnt out Britain* on BBC 2 on 25 February 2004, the cost to the government was described as being *three and a half billion pounds per annum*.)

Unbalanced intakes of food and drink are playing their part too. We might speculate that the mother is drinking to avoid or assuage emotional pain and the daughter is getting caught up in the pressures to be thin and to be perceived as attractive. Perhaps she is angry, too, with her mother at having to move schools at a vulnerable age.

One of the symptoms of these stresses is recurring headaches. Vulnerable to the inconsistencies of access to the NHS, she is relieved to gain instant help from the Alternative Medical Centre. There, thanks to time and individual attention, relief of her symptoms is acquired and she leaves feeling better. However, these feelings are not the whole story; they are concealing the facts that both she and her daughter have problems to solve – their drinking and dietary habits, for a start. Further, in her relief at instant help, she is vulnerable to not asking questions about the qualifications of the therapist and embarking on what may be an expensive series of appointments.

Part of being a good parent is knowing when and how to 'let go' of children. If this mother is grieving the loss of the child she once knew, she might be trying to hold on to that child and inadvertently conveying the message not to grow up. The girl seems to be receiving other ideas, such as the importance of being slim in order to be accepted and sexually attractive. What might be the consequences of the loss of the father to this household of two females?

We live in a sexualised society. What are the effects of this on our psychological health? Think of how our bodies change as we get older, for example. Think of the fact that we have no control over the anatomical structure we inherit at birth. How many people feel that their bodies and their personalities match? Inside every fat person (who is often burdened with having to pretend to be jollier than they feel because of notions that 'fat people are jolly') there is a thin person struggling to get out, we are told. Maybe inside every thin person, there is a fat person wanting to be soft and cuddly. It is politically incorrect to say 'fat people'. We find ourselves using euphemisms in everyday life, such as 'larger ladies'; but in a clinical context we may have to work with the consequences of obesity. The Body Shop produced a booklet in 1997[1] referring to a study that asked women to report how they felt after looking at glossy magazines for no more than three minutes. Seventy per cent of the sample reported feelings of depression. Until recently, the pressure to conform to a media stereotype was only applied to women. But now men find their sense of masculinity threatened, if they are not wearing 'designer' labels over a six-pack musculature, leaving a trail of pungent aftershave in their wake as they strut down the high street. And, as we all know, it is not easy to strut under a British climate.

Personal and professional development

1 Reflect on your experience of mother/daughter relationships during teenage years. What sort of role did your father/stepfather play?
2 Evaluate the impact of food and drink in your life, in terms of the balance between physiological and psychological needs.
3 Research the literature on stress, headaches, migraines and evidence-based medicine (EBM) relating to the long-term effects of migraine-relief medication.
4 In terms of health service policy, how can the safety of orthodox medicine be adopted by the complementary system so that vulnerable patients do not get treatment from inappropriately qualified personnel?
5 The alternative therapist is different from NHS personnel, in her frank disclosure of her own similar problems. To what extent would greater disclosure 'humanise' medical systems? What are the risks?
6 If you were nursing an anorexic teenager, how would you handle the mother/parents?
7 List the number of losses that this mother is experiencing. How would you counsel her through them?
8 Do you think it would be a good idea for a practice nurse to set up a self-help group for people (mixed men and women, or women only?) struggling with image-consciousness?
9 This woman's symptoms were healed by good listening skills. Reflect on your use of listening in your work.
10 Imagine you are running a health promotion campaign. How would you limit the pressures from the media relating to food and drink?

Useful tip
Mind your mind ... and remember what it was like to be a teenager.

Reference

1 The Body Shop (1997) *Full Voice.* Issue one. The Body Shop, Littlehampton, Sussex (in-house publication).

D is for Dignity

'I've always suffered with a weak chest. I was also born premature (only three pounds at birth) and my doctor says that's why I've had to have so many operations on my nose. I've lost count of the number of times I've had to be admitted for polyps to be removed. Have you ever had polyps? Have you ever had a hot wire pushed up your nose, halfway into your brain?

I can go on for so long and then my breathing gets worse, my chest feels congested and the snoring is so bad that I'm sure it contributed to the breakdown of my marriage. Now I am in my late 50s and I have completely lost my sense of smell. The ENT surgeon and his staff don't have the time to discuss the effects of this loss, and as a fellow professional, I respect that fact. People think noses are funny, and, as my wife said, it would be much worse to lose your sight or your hearing. But for me, what kept me going in a difficult job and marriage was the Wine Tasting Circle.

It's the loss of dignity that goes with the sudden nosebleeds that can happen at any time. I am a headmaster of a major secondary school with a top league rating and yet, regrettably, I am getting increasingly anxious about speaking in public. At the last parents' evening, I had just welcomed everybody into the hall when a rush of blood gushed all over my shirt and tie. I had no choice but to leave the room immediately. My deputy took over and she is a very ambitious person and somehow the word has got round that I am going to take early retirement. My job *is* my life. I have no intention at all of leaving the profession early. I have made this school what it is. I have great plans for its future. There have been rumours that these nosebleeds are caused by high blood pressure, which is not true. I used to carry a freshly laundered white handkerchief for such emergencies but, since my wife left, it is not easy to look as smart as I used to do. Even the garden looks a mess. I have always taken pride in a perfect lawn. I mowed, my wife clipped. Now I have to do the edges myself.

I was irritated last week when I had to take an hour out of school for a tetanus injection. I expected the doctor to do it but the receptionist informed me that nurses do this kind of thing now. The young nurse looked familiar but I could not place her. After I had rolled my sleeve up, I suddenly felt very anxious. Just as she jabbed me, I realised that I had taught her years before and had had some very awkward meetings with her parents. The trouble was

I could not remember anything else. I wanted to get out as quickly as possible, but she took control by saying that we might as well run through one or two other health checks while I was there. Before I knew it, she had me talking about all sorts of private things. She even had me admit to feeling down about my age and the threats to my career. Then she announced that she thought that she knew me from somewhere and had I been her teacher? I had no choice but to tell the truth and she started laughing in a really unnerving way. I found myself blushing as if I were a child. I did not know where to put myself.

When I thought about the incident later, I realised that I had missed a chance to talk to somebody sympathetic about the loss of my marriage. But I couldn't face making another appointment just in case she had told the receptionist about how strict I had been. You see, nobody knows I've been shy all my life.'

Psychological issues

In this scenario, we have a middle-aged man who is used to being in a job which gives him control. But he is facing several uncontrollable things:

- the ageing process (dwindling senses)
- unpredictable nosebleeds
- his wife leaving him
- his deputy threatening his position
- a sudden shift in the power balance when the nurse gets him to open up about his feelings.

We are always on dangerous ground if we assume we know what makes somebody tick (especially in the clinical setting). But we can ask questions:

- What might be the long-term effects of being born prematurely?
- Could the helplessness of the very small baby be translated into a drive-to-survive?
- Was he attracted to a job that gives him power and control over others as a compensation for feeling small inside?
- Chest weaknesses such as breathlessness are frightening; is he over-compensating by 'puffing himself up' psychologically too?

It is not surprising that a loss of dignity is a dread in his mind. Feeling laughed at is an uncomfortable experience at any time, but the more so for this character, in this surgery, with this 'young' nurse.

Further, he is vulnerable to middle-aged memory loss, his awareness that he cannot recall this ex-pupil's name. Predictably, he can recall the (painful) emotional connotation in his memory (tricky parent interview), but not the detail. For teachers to say 'I don't know' is as hard as it is for medical staff to say 'I don't care'.

Note how jobs can infect our identities. We can become so wrapped up in what we do that we can confuse this with who we are (*see* the Introduction re: doing/being/having).

Professional boundaries and expectations about the changing nature of disclosures are also issues here. Note how the headmaster does *not* expect 'sensitivity-type-discussions' with the ENT team and is therefore perhaps taken aback when this nurse provides holistic care.

Personal and professional development

1 Loss of dignity may not seem to be a particularly big loss. Loss of life, loss of a limb, loss of a friend are more serious on the scale of relative losses. People who are in positions of power and authority may therefore be more vulnerable to this sort of loss.

   How do you think this affects healthcare professionals when they themselves become ill?

   To what extent do you *identify* with your job? Do threats to your role feel like personal affronts?

2 Reflect on times when you have felt embarrassed at work? How did you cope? Does wearing a uniform/name badge help you to feel confident?

3 Research the literature on authority,[1] obedience and control.

4 Loss of a sense is serious. We usually think that we have five senses but there is the sixth sense – the proprioceptive sense or sense of having a body. 'The Disembodied Lady' in Oliver Sacks' book, makes interesting reading.[2] Sight and hearing are the most feared losses, of course. It is not just the loss of the sense of smell which hurts this patient, but the reminder of the ageing process, exacerbated in this scenario by the age differential between himself and the nurse.

   Do you think the NHS is right to consider reducing access to some services for the very elderly on the grounds of rationalisation of resources?

5 Reflect on your need for control.

6 Repeated operations under anaesthetic have probably increased this man's fear of the loss of control. What measures are taken by theatre teams to mitigate such anxiety?

7 Put yourself in the shoes of the practice nurse. This scenario raises issues about disclosure. What are the advantages and disadvantages of her saying that she was taught by him?

8 In what ways might the nurse follow up this consultation?

9 Loss of dignity, through nosebleeds, may remind us of embarrassing experiences that bodily fluids cause (e.g. incontinence, menstruation, drooling, crying). Adults often apologise if they break down crying. How do you use the sense of touch?

10 We can easily overlook the fact that when patients visit surgeries or hospitals, they are out of their own 'territory'. We may be so used to being healthcare professionals, to being part of that group, in that institution, that we forget that it is our duty to receive them with skills of hospitality. How can health services do this better, from letters to patients, to the first encounter between the patient and the professional?

References

1 Milgram S (1974) *Obedience to Authority.* Pinter and Martin, London.

2 Sacks O (1985) *The Man Who Mistook His Wife for a Hat.* Picador, London.

E is for Energy

'There were four children in our family – my brother, me, my mum, my dad. They were the kids, always arguing and threatening to split up. They had high expectations of us as they'd both wanted to be doctors but had only got the grades to be dentists. So they packed us off to boarding school at seven years of age, telling us that if we worked hard we could become consultants.

Marcus got a scholarship to Cambridge but I lost my way in the sixth form, falling in love with one of the teachers. Time went by, and Marcus and I shared a flat in London while he did his hospital training. He was out every night having a good time. Meanwhile, I was starting to feel more and more tired. At first he was helpful and told me to have blood tests but they didn't show anything up and he lost interest. I just spent the days sleeping in front of the telly. Then, one night I got in the way of one of his many girlfriends and the next morning he told me to 'get a life or get out of the flat'. I went wandering around the streets of London wondering what to do. I saw so many poor people. I could not face going back home to Cheshire, so I started working in a hostel for the homeless. One of the guys there became a good friend so I let him use Marcus's flat while he was on a skiing trip (aiming to achieve the quadruple twisting triple back somersault).

"I work hard and I play hard", he shouted, snatching the keys to the flat, on his return. "I suggest you both do the same!" I had no choice but to return home.

"Tired Andrew? Exhausted? Don't be such a nancy-boy!" My dad shouted.

"Why can't you be like Marcus?" Mum whined.

"You want to get yourself a job! Join the army, like your grandad did!"

"Yes. Your dad's right. If you can't make it as a medic, then you'd better become a Major. ... Look, Geoffrey, he's whimpering again. Do something about it!"

"It's never too late to become a dentist, lad. Your mother and I only want you to be happy ... like Marcus."

"We only ever wanted you to be happy. And there's no shame, nowadays, in just being a dentist you know. We make more money and you can always call yourself an oral surgeon."

The next thing that happens is mum persuades dad to persuade Nikki, his hygienist, to ask her dad (who's a neurologist) to put me in a scanner. (They're willing to pay to find out what's wrong with me.)

Marcus tells them to save their money and he pronounces his diagnoses. I have TATT (tired all the time) or ME (myalgic encephalitis) or chronic fatigue syndrome and I should see a consultant specialising in metabolic disorders.

When I got back to London I went to a GP instead. She was very good and had just been on a course about ME. She advised me to do some gentle exercise every day and to remind myself that it was probably 'all in the mind'. I made another appointment to see her because she was such a good listener, but the next time it was a locum who said I was probably pushing myself too much and should relax. On the way home I saw an alternative health centre and bought some 'energising crystals'.

Months went by. London was grey and rainy. Christmas was coming and I was spending the whole time watching videos in the attic at the flat. Marcus had said that I could stay there if I kept out of his way. He had been telling me that I was probably a secret depressive like mum and offered to pay for a series of private sessions with a psychiatrist he knew in Hampstead. He said I could make a real contribution to research, as I was such a complex case.

I was thinking of hanging myself with Marcus's stethoscope when he returned from Cheshire at the beginning of January. Something had changed in him. He was quieter. He had had a health scare himself, back trouble, linked to his skiing trip. The next few months were better between us and gradually I pulled myself out of the black hole.

Now, five years on, I am getting my life together. I'm training as a nurse. I never saw a psychiatrist. I'd rather have had ME than 'depression' with the stigma that goes with it.'

Psychological issues

We are presented with a dysfunctional family. Notice how:

- the parents behave like children
- the lines of communication are fuzzy – mum speaking for dad, dad speaking for mum, younger son being spoken about as if he is not there
- sibling rivalry is exacerbated by people telling the younger brother that he should be more like Marcus, his older brother
- there are inappropriate expectations.

Loss of energy is the presenting problem and the young man is offered *inconsistent advice:*

- blood tests
- resting
- exercise
- neurological scanning
- psychiatry
- metabolic disorder consultation.

So he buys 'energising crystals' and spends his days watching television.

Labels and acronyms play a part in this scenario. TATT or ME, neither sounds particularly attractive, and what do they mean? Notice how even though the patient is going on to train as a nurse, he is wary of carrying a psychiatric label himself.

Energy is probably one of *the most intangible* losses, from the viewpoint of the clinical observer. How can we read the energy levels in a person? We can't. We can 'read' faces and body language, but in a 10-minute consultation in primary care, how can we accurately assess the degree to which the person in front of us is less energetic than usual. If we listen carefully, we may get some idea but we must be wary of assumptions and conclusions.

Loss of emotional health might be a good description of the loss experienced by this young man, or is it more a case of 'lack'? We do not get the impression that emotional health was there in the first place. Think of the following feelings:

- lonely
- unhappy
- miserable
- sad
- desperate
- envious
- tired.

Do you think they can really be matched by psychiatric diagnoses?

Do you think psychiatric labels help?

Do you think emotional problems fit comfortably with a medical model? (You might like to check the literature on neuroscience to see how far the mapping of brain cells/emotions has progressed.)

Is it not more appropriate to apply a 'needs model' for people in emotional pain? – What does she or he need? instead of What is wrong with her or him?

Feelings of loneliness may be expressed by patients if they feel safe enough (and if there is enough time).

'Loneliness' will not be found on a sick-note; a prescription will not be available to cure it. To what extent do you think it is an inevitable outcome in a society where broken relationships, in families and elsewhere, have become the norm?

'I had no choice ...'. The patient perceives himself to be 'choiceless', when in truth, as an adult, he has choice. He is expressing the common difficulty with decision making when reduced to a sense of powerlessness in the diminished condition in which he finds himself. Perhaps he presents with loss of energy rather than depression, because he does not want to connect with his mother who is described as a 'secret depressive'?

Personal and professional development

1 *Acronyms** Do you ever feel threatened when presented with an acronym you don't understand? In this example, TATT and ME do not have positive connotations, do they? One sounds tatty and the other, selfish. Reflect on the impact of acronyms on patients. We take for granted commonly used terms like CHD (congestive heart disease) and RTA (road traffic accident), and they may be necessary professional shorthand, but to an anxious patient they can sound threatening. How do you use acronyms in clinical practice?

2 *Inconsistencies* This patient is burdened with conflicting advice. EBM (evidence-based medicine) is the move to secure greater certainty in diagnosis and treatment. But intangible suffering like this, when a patient presents with *loss of energy* is difficult to place within any clear clinical context. What measures could be taken, within clinical teams, to limit the damage done by inconsistent advice?

3 Inconsistencies, nationwide, in access to care are a serious problem. What should the government do about this?

4 Have you tried 'energising crystals'? What do you think of CAM (complementary and alternative medicine)?

5 *Parents* These parents are made-to-measure for the sake of this scenario, the aim of which is to show the psychological cost of unrealistic expectations. There is a danger of re-presenting the argument – 'let's blame parents' for our emotional problems.

---

*PVS (persistent vegetative state) sounds better as an acronym whereas SAD (seasonal affective disorder), for example, is better the other way round.

> But they were fucked up in their turn
> By fools in old-style hats and coats,
> Who half the time were soppy-stern
> And half at one another's throats.
>
> *This Be the Verse* – the second stanza

Philip Larkin[1] is referring to the fact that even though 'they fuck you up, your mum and dad', they too had parents who may have 'fucked' them up.

6 Three issues emerge from this example:

- the effect of diagnostic labelling on perceptions
- the stigma of mental illness
- the long-term effect of poor parenting.

Reflect on your experience in this context. To what extent do you think parents are responsible for the emotional development of their children?

7 In what small ways do you think you can contribute to changing the thinking in health from splitting people into physical and mental aspects?

8 Various statistics are quoted about the amount of people who enjoy 'secure attachments' in childhood. Bowlby (a psychoanalyst) in the 1950s suggested that 60% of mothers do a very good job, the corollary being that 40% do not.[2] Oliver James, a clinical psychologist, puts forward a 50–50 split, going on to describe the less fortunate half as being clingers, avoidants or wobblers.[3] What do you make of this terminology?

9 If you were to care for the younger brother in this scenario, where would you start?

10 How far do you think medical training encourages toughness at the expense of sensitivity?

Useful tip
Mind your mind. Check ... are you becoming tough at the expense of sensitivity?

References

1 Larkin P (1988) *Collected Poems*. Faber and Faber, London.

2 Bowlby (1953) *Child Care and the Growth of Love*. Pelican, London.

3 James O (2002) *They Fuck You Up*. Bloomsbury, London.

F is for Fear
(of the loss of . . .)

'I am one of those lucky women. I have it all – a wonderful partner, two brilliant kids and a big circle of friends. It helps being American and married to a realtor. I started out as a model, moved into PR and then, when the girls started school I decided I didn't just want to be a mom or a career woman any more. So I guess I'm a 'lady-who-lunches'. I have breakfast out every day too, and most evenings I'm at a dinner party raising funds for charity. It's the American Dream made real, but in the UK with all the quaint stuff that goes with it. I look after myself and I like to go on the internet to check out the supplements. Have you heard of takionic energy?

I didn't understand all the science behind it but it said "Fluids in your body cannot effectively transport oxygen and nutrients to your cells or remove toxins from them due to large water clusters. This causes your cells to age faster and become unhealthy. Takionic products help break up large water clusters, thereby improving assimilation of oxygen and nutrients and the removal of wastes. Cells maintain their youthful vitality and optimum health." I ordered their takionic mattress straight away. It was a little expensive (£1000), but anything that can give you a boost has to be worth it. And sure enough, my long-standing problem of insomnia was healed – overnight.

But then I started getting these weird allergic reactions. So did the girls. We had all suffered with our skin at one time or the other and, frankly, I was disappointed with the local surgery when I rang up. They said we had to go through the GP to see a dermatologist and that there wasn't an appointment until the end of the week. I was getting palpitations even though I had given up caffeine ages ago. My father died from a heart condition and by the end of the phone call I had developed chest pains and I felt dizzy. I took a precautionary aspirin in case it was a stroke. Mandy-Sue said she felt dizzy too and I thought it wouldn't do her any harm either to take an aspirin. So I drove down to the surgery to book the whole family in for a check-up.

The receptionist did not give me the attention I expected. After I had strained my neck trying to talk to her through the small window in reception, after I had handed her the details of the takionic products we had been trying, she said, without smiling "Anything else?" She sounded like a shop assistant and I was just about to get assertive when I saw a notice on the wall warning patients about abusing staff. I guess I really wanted to say something about the system abusing the individual. Just then my mobile went off and it was Donna-Lee saying she had come home from school early with a red itchy rash all over her body. I told her to meet me at the surgery. The receptionist suddenly discovered a cancelled appointment on her screen.

Although the doctor looked at her watch during the consultation, at least she got the right diagnosis for Donna-Lee – *Pityriasis rosea*, a nervous skin reaction due to the pressures of exams, she said. She offered to give me a quick check-up while I was there. She took my blood pressure (with one of those historic sphygmomanometers), asked me a lot of 'lifestyle' questions and suggested that I could do with more exercise and a healthier diet. As she gave me extra time I started to unwind a little and I told her how much we spent, as a family, on internet products to secure our health. I explained that I had this morbid fear of growing old and looking old. There was something really nice about this doctor. She pointed out to me that there is more to life than a 'lifestyle'. It's something we all know, I think, but you can easily lose sight of the spiritual things when you are caught up in bringing up a family and doing charity work. She said the practice nurse was starting up a self-help group for women who are image-conscious, and my daughter, and I signed up there and then for the monthly meetings.

When we got home I talked to my husband. He agreed that the NHS isn't adequate for our family needs and that we would go private from now on. We'd tried to support the state system. I'd raised money at charity balls for the local hospital but when it's your own family, you can't be too careful.'

Psychological issues

This scenario represents the hidden costs of 'having it all'. The woman is fearful about losing her health, to the point of hypochondria. Her children are picking up on this anxiety and one is saying she feels dizzy like her mother. The other has a rash, which may be linked to anxiety about exams. The doctor identifies a weight problem as a real physical problem and suggests that the woman and her daughters may be caught up in the pressures of a modern lifestyle (which tends to value youth more than experience).

There is the cultural difference in her expectations of the NHS compared with her American experience. She expects to get an immediate appointment and instant access to a specialist.

The issue of getting medical information from the internet is a source of concern for healthcare professionals, partly because it erodes the power base of medicine. The scientific basis for the product is questionable. Do you think her problem with insomnia might have been eased due to the placebo effect?

The cost of her lifestyle is a theme in this scenario. It would seem to be contributing to a spiritual emptiness. Her demanding approach in reception might have given her the short-term solution of an appointment, but it is at the cost of alienating the receptionist.

The doctor is seen to look at her watch at first, but gives time to this woman to discuss the wider issues behind the appointment. The term 'malingerer' may be used in general practice. To what extent do you think that hypochondriacs take up unnecessary time?

Receptionists can be much maligned by patients because they may be perceived as the gatekeepers to the system. This one did not smile and, protected by the barrier of the small window, might convey a further inaccessibility to an already frustrated patient. But it is worth remembering the pressures experienced by receptionists and other administrators in primary healthcare. Is the current provision of 'protected learning time', one afternoon a month for training, the best way to do staff development?

This mother is giving her daughter an aspirin because she is taking one too. Is she conditioning her daughter to rely on medication for symptom relief when the symptoms may not be real? She is also vulnerable to an array of dubious internet products in her quest for eternal youth.

Finally, the family decide to go private because 'you cannot be too careful about your own health'.

Personal and professional development

1 Imagine a meeting with a patient who seems to be a hypochondriac. How far would you accept them for the anxiety they experience and how far would you challenge them for the time they are taking up?

2 Reflect on body image and the pressures to look young. Would it be a good idea for a practice nurse to set up a self-help group for men and women (or women only?) to support each other against the pressures of the media to look a certain way?

3 Where do your loyalties lie – in the public or private health system? What is the moral argument for equal access to healthcare irrespective of income or lifestyle? How far is it realistic to expect as much individual attention under the NHS as in private consultations? And how important is 'attention'? Should primary care operate a system which balances the quality of time given with the quantity demanded by patients? For example, should

each patient have an annual review of the demands they have made on the system and a meeting to negotiate access in the forthcoming year?

4 Think about the overlap between physical and spiritual needs. How comfortable are you about discussing intangible things such as religious or spritual matters?

5 What are you most scared of losing?

6 What is the most frightening moment so far in your professional career?

7 How do you react to fear? Do you tend to favour 'fight', 'flight' or 'freeze'?

8 How do you support your colleagues when they are scared?

9 Do you use humour to ease the tensions? Can it be misplaced with some patients?

10 To what extent do you think the UK is moving towards the American system of healthcare?

Useful tip

Feeling old? Stick a Post-It© with the number 90 on your mirror. Then, when you look at yourself, you will see how young you look by comparison. The psychology of expectations is very powerful.

Even more useful tip

It is not how you look that matters, but how you are.

G is for Guilt
(about the loss of . . .)

'I never thought I'd do it. I never thought I'd be a mother who walked out on her children. It all happened years ago and my son and daughter are grown up and doing very well in London. They are also in good relationships so any idea that there are long-term effects of what I did, I can forget. I say that, but there isn't a day that goes by when I don't feel some guilt about what I did. The social stigma has been with me and I have just limited myself to mixing either with single people or couples who don't have children. It's not fair really; men who stop being fathers are almost the norm these days, but a woman who leaves her children when they are under the age of 10 is not acceptable.

I had moved south when we split up but I drove north every weekend to see them. One late Friday night on a rainy motorway in November, I had an accident. I crashed into the back of a Mercedes. I suffered shock and bruising and had to go to A&E. They took all my details and when I cried about the children, they were very sympathetic. But later on, I'm sure I saw two members of staff talking about me, shaking their heads and when I was discharged, one definitely gave me a funny look.

Apart from some minor digestive problems, my health has held up well over the years until bowel trouble started. I went to the doctor but he was very reassuring, suggesting that I needed to improve my diet and take more care of myself. When I left the surgery that day I thought of all the questions I had wanted to ask but didn't like to. They were short-staffed. The practice nurse was off with stress herself, I think, and the doctor was doing the injections as well as fitting everybody in to their appointment slots. Then I noticed blood in my stools and saw a different doctor at the practice. He said we'd sort it out together and got on the phone to arrange for tests at the hospital. But there was some sort of problem. He said "Can you manage for a few more days?" I felt obliged to say 'yes' and immediately regretted it.

A few weeks later it was my son's wedding. I had to meet up with my ex-husband for the first time in several years. We both wanted it to be a good occasion. But the stress played havoc with my digestion. I had to wear incontinence pads in case of an accident. My ex-husband had a new girlfriend, a nurse practitioner. She was a lot of fun and I felt envious when I saw her chatting comfortably to my son's wife. Later, after we'd all had a few drinks, we got talking and she asked me about my health. I told her a bit about the problem. She laughed and said "You don't want to have a colostomy bag at your age! You're still quite young, really". I don't think I had ever thought so far ahead. Perhaps I had blocked it all out. The day the photographs came back coincided with the day I was due at the hospital for the tests.

I now help run the survivors' group at the local hospital. I have met so many people who have come through cancer. They all believe that having a positive frame of mind helped them. The quality of care is the best when you get cancer. I suppose that's because with heart disease and strokes, the patients could at least have done something to prevent themselves getting ill. Couldn't they?'

Psychological issues

This woman is suffering from guilt about the loss of her children through divorce. She is aware that men who leave are seen as being part of the norm, whereas a mother who leaves her children carries a stigma.

We might *speculate* that her 'digestive problems' link psychologically with guilt, in that guilt reduces self-esteem and may contribute to an unwillingness to nurture oneself.

She believes that some staff in A&E have commented negatively about her after her accident and after they have kindly supported her about the children. We might say that it is just in her mind, that anyone after an accident is in a vulnerable state and therefore prone to misperceptions. However, it is possible that the staff discussed her and yet their shaking of heads might have been in sympathy rather than criticism. 'Body language' is very powerful. Our gestures, facial expressions and tone of voice matter in the clinical area.

The first doctor is pleasantly reassuring and useful in reminding this woman to look after herself. However as soon as she is out of the surgery, she thinks of all the questions that she wished that she had asked. This is very common, thinking of questions after the consultation. Reassurance itself, though comforting, can be dangerous if, as in this case, the clinician misses the problem.

The second doctor who tries to get her an appointment at the hospital for bowel tests is in a difficult situation because of being on the telephone. However, asking the closed question 'Can you manage …?', persuades this patient to say 'Yes'. Also, suggesting that they are going to sort the problem together (patients as partners) may or may not inspire confidence. Some patients want to be treated in this way. Others may want the traditional approach of putting their trust in the doctor's expertise.

The fear of wearing a colostomy bag is an extra psychological burden.

The bowels are an area of the body about which people are often embarrassed. The fear of being dirty, the fear of having a soiling accident, the indignity of wearing incontinence pads, the fear of an enema may all contribute to increasing the risk of not asking questions in this area. Examining one's own stools for blood is unlikely to be a pleasant experience. Is there a place here for health promotion? Literature (often of an alarmist sort) was produced in the 1980s about safe sex. Could we do the same for our bowels?

Do you think that people could look after their hearts and brains better, whereas there is less responsibility for getting cancer? As we move towards times where the responsibility we take for our health may be rewarded (or otherwise, as in the suggestion of a 'fat tax'), what do you think are the moral justifications for rationalisation in the NHS?

Personal and professional development

1 Reflect on your experience of guilt in your personal and professional life.
2 We are responsible *to* one another, not *for* one another. Do you agree?
3 Do you regularly reflect on your 'body language'? Do you know if you have mannerisms? Have you sought feedback from colleagues on how you come across in the way in which you speak – the pace, tone and clarity of your voice? We are often more anxious about our accents, but the pace and tone will convey emotion, and without clarity we may just as well not speak at all. When we are anxious, we may sound impatient or even angry. When we are unsure of ourselves, the volume of our voices may either soften to the point of inaudibility or become too loud.
4 Have you observed incidents where professionals have believed themselves to be out of the range of the patients, and behaved unprofessionally, either by whispering about patients or relatives, or looking at them in a negative way?
5 The practice nurse is understood to be off work due to stress. What sort of stresses are unique to practice nurses? One thing you might consider for a new practice nurse is the adjustment that she or he has to make to a more isolated situation than teamwork in either the community or in hospital. How far do feelings of isolation affect your practice?
6 There are open and closed questions, and each must be used in the right way and at the right time. Are you confident that you know the difference and use these appropriately?
7 The patient, on one occasion, thinks of what she wanted to ask only after leaving the surgery. What are the best ways to avoid this common difficulty?

8 How comfortable are you with talking about bowels? Do you find you cover any embarrassment by the use of humour? The medical profession often uses an earthy sort of humour, which may ease tensions amongst colleagues, but could it be inappropriate with some patients?
9 If you were to help this woman from an holistic angle, where would you begin?
10 Would you feel differently about giving emotional support to a 'guilty man' than to a 'guilty woman'?

Useful tip
We are responsible *to* one another not *for* one another (unless in the role of a parent or caring professional). There are, therefore, boundaries to be drawn around the corrosive effects of long-term guilt.

H is for Husband

'A salmon-hatchery manager from the Kyle of Lochalsh sent me a photo-graph of his erection. That was just two years after my husband had died. It had been so difficult trying to get a social life going in my 50s that I had ended up answering one of those adverts in the personal column of a national newspaper. My husband and I had been together since the age of 16; we had done everything together and so we didn't really have friends. I was so lonely without him. I answered two adverts actually, and when I tried to stop the other man (a solicitor from Cornwall) from turning up on my doorstep, he told me that I didn't know what I was missing as his was nine and a half inches long.

I decided to take up an interest. I joined the local sports club and gradually began to meet people and to enjoy the increased fitness that went with it. Then one day my back went. I had never had trouble before and I thought I knew how to look after it. I put a hot water bottle on it that night, but the following day I was in so much pain I could hardly make it to the phone to ring NHS Direct. The nurse was informative but brisk. She told me to take both painkillers (paracetamol) and an anti-inflammatory (ibuprofen). She also said that I should have put a bag of frozen peas on it first and then warm my back up the next day. There wasn't time to explain to her that I was unable to bend down to get in the freezer to reach the peas. I nearly cried and she said "Are you all right?" The next few days were very frustrating. On one occasion I very nearly didn't make it to the toilet from my bed. The nurse had warned me that I might get some stomach trouble with the ibuprofen and maybe that was what triggered a bit of diarrhoea. I only had a kitchen broom to use as an aid to get me into a standing position. As I pushed myself off the bed, using my thigh muscles I think I probably strained a muscle in my leg. If I could have sat down and cried, I would have. My back went into spasm and all the feelings of isolation came back. I was really scared of being on my own. Supposing I got stuck and nobody found me? I thought that I had been through the hard work of grief but anger threatened to overwhelm me. How could Tony have died so suddenly? Why didn't the ambulance men do more to save him? We had been in bed and he was sleeping beside me when all of a sudden he shuddered and that was it. I rang 999 and they tried to resuscitate him but it was too late. If only I had known how to give the kiss of life.

When my back got better, I didn't really want to risk any damage to it again, so I gave up my membership at the club. I started getting low and a neighbour who was a student nurse suggested that I should stop turning the anger against myself. She had been very kind in the first few months after Tony's death, but the way she said it, she sounded as if she was blaming me. She reminded me that it was five years on and that I *should* be rebuilding my life by now, getting out and meeting new people. How could I tell her about the postal erection? Insomnia got worse and I seemed to be getting more and more accident-prone, just little things like stumbling but I decided it would be best not to learn to drive. I had planned to get a car to use the freedom that my neighbour said I *should* enjoy.

Things came to a head one Easter. Everyone else was with everyone else. Even on the television, there were holiday programmes showing people together, romantic films or 'family' entertainment. My husband and I had not been able to have children. He would not talk about it and I suppose I carried that particular lack alone. I still had the paracetamol in the house. I was tempted to take the lot. What's a woman got to live for after the menopause, anyway?

I rang the surgery and the out-of-hours number was given to me. I felt so guilty. I wasn't ill. I was just desperate. Within a few hours a foreign doctor came to my door. He said he would assess me. There was something about that word 'assess'. It made me feel judged. I have probably never forgiven myself for my husband's death and I just started to cry. The doctor was very kind and took my hand. He asked me all about Tony and I think it was the first time I had had such a good listener. I did find his accent hard to understand, but it didn't really matter because he wasn't doing much of the talking. But when he said he had to go, I felt abandoned all over again. He suggested I see my GP immediately after Easter with a view to getting an appointment with a psychiatrist. I was hurt because I'm not mad but sad. My GP was good. She put me on Seroxat© and Evorel© (HRT − hormone replacement therapy). After a while I realised I was better with just 10 mg of Seroxat©, even though the therapeutic dose is 20 mg. I never told the doctor.'

Psychological issues

This woman is suffering the loneliness that follows after the death of somebody very close. Her marriage has been a long one without the necessity to have friends, so she is even more isolated. This loneliness has made her vulnerable and she has acted out of character, it seems, by answering some adverts in the 'lonely hearts' column of a newspaper. Perhaps she is thinking that she can replace one marriage for another? It is more likely that she only knows the marital state as a source of company because we get the impression that she was deeply attached to her husband and that they were 'childhood sweethearts'. The shock of the sexualised correspondence has persuaded her to join the sports club.

However, she hurts her back, which reinforces feelings of isolation. She perceives the voice of the nurse at NHS Direct as being 'brisk' and becomes tearful when told how she should have dealt with the back injury. The nurse, limited by being on a telephone line, asks if she is all right (which clearly she isn't). There isn't the time to explore the emotional problem in depth.

She now experiences frustration and the fear of having an accident by not making it to the toilet. Suddenly her frustration ignites the anger about her loss, which she had not let herself feel during the 'hard work of grief'. Regrets pour in as she re-lives, in her mind, the night her husband died. It was a sudden death. She had no preparation. The ambulance men should have done more. She should have known how to give the kiss of life.

Fearful for her back, she retreats into herself. A neighbour who is a student nurse wants to help and suggests that she is turning the anger against herself. Trying to help, she suggests that the patient learns to drive. But the advice is perceived as pressure because of the term 'should' and what might have been a helpful dialogue nosedives into distorted communication.

Easter arrives. It is a vulnerable time. The patient perceives 'everybody else' to be with 'everybody else'. Loneliness and feelings of despair increase. She feels worthless because she is menopausal. She is attracted to the para-cetamol. She is reluctant to seek help because she sees herself as not being ill but being desperate. The foreign doctor comes to see her and listens to her story about Tony, her late husband. He takes her hand. But then he, too, has to leave and she has feelings of abandonment again. She is hurt by his use of the word 'assess' and by his suggestion of a referral to a psychiatrist, perceiving the latter to be a diagnosis of madness (not sadness).

Finally, her GP uses a pharmacological intervention in the form of Seroxat (an antidepressant) and Evorel (HRT patches). She discovers the right dose for her needs but does not tell the doctor.

Personal and professional development

1 Reflect on your experience of the loss of somebody close. In this example, feelings of sadness, anger and isolation are apparent, as is guilt too, for not being able to do more to save her husband's life. What sort of feelings have you experienced?

2 Review the literature on stage theories of grief:

- numbness
- denial
- anger
- bargaining
- depression.

What are the advantages and disadvantages of such theories?

3 Sudden death, as in this case, is arguably harder to cope with because the mind does not have time to prepare itself for the loss. The ambulance men who attended her husband would not have had time to stay with her at that point. She had no children and no need of friends due to the very close nature of her marriage. How could the health service have helped her at the point of crisis? If help had been available then, do you think that she would have been able to come to terms with the loss sooner?

4 'Should' is a difficult term in emotional advice because it can convey criticism. If a patient is vulnerable, this can exacerbate the feelings of in-adequacy. The nurse at NHS Direct uses the term in the context of clinical advice, which is slightly different (i.e. she should have used the cold compress before the hot one) but because of the nature of the patient's feelings, this brief conversation is unsatisfactory, ending with the nurse asking a closed question, 'Are you all right?', when she isn't. Would it be a good idea to have a branch of NHS Direct available for consultations specifically offering emotional support?

5 Advice carries authority. What is the difference between giving advice as a professional in a clinical context and giving it as a neighbour? How much difference does it make, the fact that the neighbour is a student nurse?

5 Back injuries limit mobility, at least temporarily. Loss of mobility can induce feelings of isolation. Feelings of isolation have led to the fear of abandonment and a reminder of the sudden death of her husband. Easter arrives and with it, feelings of despair. The emergency doctor holds her hand. What do you make of this?

6 *Seeing herself as not ill but desperate* supports the view that the public tend to perceive the health service as being for purely physical problems only. Fearful that the referral to a psychiatrist suggests that she is mad rather than sad reminds us that psychiatry in many people's minds is firmly associated with notions of madness ... and the fear of being labelled 'mad'. Could you invent a health promotion campaign that educates the public about *holistic* medicine but without raising expectations too much?

7 We use terms like 'assess' as part of professional language. In this scenario, the vulnerable woman, on the point of considering taking an

overdose of paracetamol, interprets assessment as judgement. Are there ways round this?

8 What are the advantages and disadvantages, physically and psychologically of taking HRT?

9 How would you help this patient now?

10 There are an increasing number of healthcare professionals in the NHS from other countries, other cultures. What might be some of the implications of this for patients?

I is for Independence

'Independence has been the most important thing in my life, particularly physical independence. I had always enjoyed pushing my body to the limit. My husband and I had met on a canoeing trip at university and from that point on we took up climbing, potholing, skiing and riding. We were always extremely safety-conscious, so falling off a bike without a helmet was the last thing I expected to happen. The last thing I remember was speeding down hill on a newly gravelled road . When I came round in the ambulance, I managed to tell them that I could not feel my legs and that was in spite of my jaw being smashed and 'looking like cornflakes', they said later. They patched up my face and did a tracheotomy and put me in the high dependency unit (HDU) of our local hospital. The doctor told my husband (who had found me in the road covered in blood) that I had a 50–50 chance of getting pneumonia. I remember getting very distressed because even though I was breathing I couldn't really tell that I was breathing because of the assistance with the breathing. They kept getting my name wrong and that upset my husband, and because we had always lived for each other, to be apart so suddenly was very traumatic. We are both research scientists and it was hell to feel that nobody appreciated our knowledge of the body and the limitations of modern medicine. At one point I had a fight with one of the nurses because she had to adjust my tracheotomy and I couldn't breathe. I just started hitting her and she got very cross and told me to stop it.

It was unbelievable that having fallen over the handlebars onto my jaw, the only thing that wasn't damaged was my brain. For six weeks, I think, I was in the HDU flat on my back. The staff seemed to want to give us what they thought everybody else liked, such as television, for example. But we had never had a television. We resented what felt like the pressure to join in, to fit in with a system of care, of dependency.

Then I was transferred to a specialist unit for spinal injuries. This was much better, much more vigorous and I was determined to regain whatever mobility I could. Rumours had collected around my husband about my future, from being wheelchair-bound forever to having some sort of limited independence. So many of the patients were too scared to do much physiotherapy, but as soon as I could I was feeding myself (in spite of having lost a section of my tongue and quite a few teeth). They got me in a wheelchair and I managed to make it to the hospital shop but it took hours and the frustration was unbearable. But I never gave in to depression. Both my mother and my sister had had it and I told my husband not to let my sister visit me. The last thing I needed was any sort of emotional scene around me. My sister was hurt by this and rang the hospital for information. The staff at the HDU were completely open but it was different at the spinal injuries unit. There was a breach of confidentiality too. The nurse I'd hit at the HDU asked my sister if we got on and when she'd said "no", the nurse had told her about the difficulties she and her staff had experienced with us.

The physiotherapy was excellent. They had me on an exercise bike as soon as they could. It's strange because my worst fear of being in a wheelchair isn't really the worst thing that can happen. It's the nerve damage in my arms and hands that is probably going to be the worst thing to deal with in the long term. I have to have my left hand in a splint at night. I am having to face surgery on my jaw in the future. At least I can manage my own double incontinence. I am determined to get an adjusted car and to go back to work within the year.

They offered me counselling and that sort of thing, but my sister used to work as some sort of counsellor and it obviously didn't do her any good. My husband visited me every day in both the HDU and the spinal unit, so in a way we're closer than ever. He adjusted the house for my return, making sure that it could be as wheelchair-friendly as possible. But on my first weekend leave I did nearly break down. Going back to the house, seeing everything as it was before the accident, seeing what I had lost and what I was losing ... but it made me even more determined to fight this 'disability' with everything I have.

The medical team are very pleased with me now. I have made what is regarded as a remarkable recovery. Scientifically speaking, I wonder just how much more healing can take place in my spinal cord. I am described as 'domestic ambulatory' in the file, but I shall achieve much more than that. I've already walked a mile on my crutches. Nobody will take my independence from me.'

Psychological issues

There are many forms of independence. In this example, we have a patient who has enjoyed physical independence and, we might assume, intellectual independence as a research scientist. But we glean that emotionally she is tied to her husband, perhaps to the extent that it limits her relationships with other people who are trying to reach out to her. Marriage can breed dependency or even a symbiosis in which each partner is dependent on the other being dependent on him or her. The sudden loss of all physical independence, the fact of having to lie on her back for weeks, the separation from her husband has pushed the two of them closer together, almost as if they are one person in the fight for recovery.

There are several issues here about communication. Graphic statements about her jaw being 'like cornflakes' after the accident are probably best kept within the limits of professional communication. Unless, of course, we are trying to reinforce this patient's 'macho' approach to sport and recovery, in which case to go from a jaw 'like cornflakes' to anything resembling a normal face could be encouraging. For the doctor to tell her husband that she had a 50–50 chance of developing pneumonia would seem to be an unnecessary piece of information. The statistic is a statement of equal odds. The fear of your wife getting pneumonia, having just been through major facial surgery and a tracheotomy, is arguably too much emotional overload. We do not know how often the staff did not get the patient's name right. Communication with patients with tracheotomies and spinal injuries (which may limit gestures too) is not likely to be easy; it is therefore advisable to err on the side of anticipating needs such as the fear and confusion of not breathing naturally.

Expectations of what makes a patient comfortable in such a limited environment cannot be assumed. Here, the offer of television is not just irritating but serves to increase the sense of loss of control of her own life, tastes and habits. However, watching television is such a cultural norm in Britain that patients who do not conform to our expectations might be perceived as unusual or even difficult. This couple is also different, coming with a 'research scientist' background to illness. As healthcare professionals, we have been warned not to use unexplained jargon, but this is the sort of case where precise terminology and complete inclusion in clinical discussions would seem to be essential.

Inconsistency between the HDU and the spinal unit regarding communication to the next of kin via the telephone is an issue here. Is the sister of the patient justified in feeling angry because she has been told not to visit, and also because she has received open information from the HDU and then unanswered questions from the spinal unit? Hospitals have to be careful about information given on the telephone. There is also the 'slight breach in confidentiality' when the nurse who has been accidentally hit by the patient tells the sister about this incident and other difficulties.

Finally, we have the rejection of the offer of counselling. It seems to be at best something for weak people and at worst something quite useless.

Personal and professional development

1 Reflect on times in your life when you have suffered the loss of independence. How did you feel?

2 In relating to others, do you see yourself as more dependable or more dependent? Why?

3 How do you feel, professionally, when patients express or show dependency on you?

4 The loss of independence for this patient is serious. It seems to be as bad as a loss of identity because of the enjoyment of physically risky sports. Bearing in mind that she does not want counselling, how would you informally help her to adjust? Is there evidence of 'denial'? We sometimes assume a critical stance towards 'patients in denial', but it is worth remembering that we may need a bit of 'denial' to give ourselves time to adjust to an accident.

5 Giving (and receiving) information is what communication is all about. Do you think that there is a sense in which we sometimes overload patients and/or their carers? Would you have told the husband about the risk of pneumonia?

6 Consistency of practice is not always achieved in the health service. Do you think the sister had a right to feel angry about the different communication in the spinal unit?

7 How far did the HDU nurse break confidentiality, do you think?

8 Where are the boundaries between 'letting off steam', gossiping and breaching confidentiality?

9 Have you ever felt your clinical skills to be rejected? Put yourselves in the shoes of the specialist spinal injuries counsellor.

10 Exceptional (for whatever reason) patients may be difficult to relate to. Reflect on the sort of patients you find hard to like.

Useful tip
Gossip hurts; if you think you have the habit of gossiping, why not decide to break it today?

J is for Job

'It's not been an easy life. I was born in the back streets of Manchester and the first thing I can remember is being put into one of those tin baths, in front of the fire, for a wash. It wasn't my mum who looked after me but my gran. My mum lived with her mum because she had nowhere else to go, being on her own with me. I had a stammer and they used to hit me for it at school, telling me I was daft. Now I'm 79 years old and I'm only just managing to live on my own with the arthritis and the angina. My wife died young with bone cancer (she was only in her 40s) and I tried one of those second wives, but it was never the same, so it was quite a relief when she left me for somebody new at the Bowling Club.

I was all right in myself when I was working. I'd always worked. I'd left school at 14 and worked in the markets heaving bags of potatoes. They tell me that that's why I'm crippled now. Then I got myself a caretaker job at the local school and I loved it. I'd been there for years until my heart started playing up. By the time they pensioned me off, I was called a 'Buildings Supervisor'. I missed the kids and I missed being what I call 'necessary'. Nobody's bothered with me now, except the ambulance driver and the district nurse.

I look forward to the weekly chat with the driver. He always asks me what I think about what's wrong with the world. And I always tell him. I've got more marbles left than the rest of the passengers. They just shuffle on and off in silence. They take me to the hospital to clean out my kidneys. They tell me I've got to have this weekly dialysis for the rest of my life. They just leave me on this bed for hours and nobody bothers with me. I can't see the point of it.

The district nurse comes on a Tuesday and she'd be all right if she didn't talk all the time. She never stops. She makes me feel like she's spying on me. I can tell they want to get me out of my own home and into sheltered accommodation, so I always take time to spruce myself up for her visits. She says she's coming to check on my heart, my mobility and my medication. That's a bit of a sore point. I can't really be bothered to take all the stuff they give me at all the right times of the day. She gets cross and I think back to being hit at school for my stammer. She writes things down about me and doesn't let me see them. I want to tell her that I used to work in a school and that must mean I've got a bit of intelligence, mustn't it?

Last time, she went on and on about this course she'd been on. Something called EBM (evidence-based medicine). I got confused. My first wife was EBM, Elizabeth Barbara Morley. I started getting upset and had a bit of an accident with myself. She got all bossy again and said I'd be better off having proper care in a proper home. Then she apologised and told me she was so rushed off her feet that she hadn't even had time to get her car serviced. I sat her down with a cup of tea and insisted that I have a quick look under the bonnet. I'd always looked after the headmaster's car when I was working. She needed her points changing, one of her tyres was nearly flat and the windscreen wipers had lost all their rubber. She was very grateful and gave me this little hug. I felt the best I'd been in years.

Next time she called, she brought me a 2000-piece jigsaw. She said it would be good therapy. EBM said so. Maybe I'm starting again with those little strokes I don't like to tell them about. I'm obviously losing my marbles. But I'm not going to let them kill me off before I get to 80 years old. It says in the papers that everyone's living to 80 nowadays. I might even try for 81.

The pain is getting worse – the arthritis. I don't let on. That second wife had all sorts of things she wanted doing to the house. And I just pushed myself to get everything done. She had new electrics, a paved patio area (with barbecue facilities) and a front porch. It looked daft on our tiny street. When I look back, that's when the chest pains started too. But I always thought it was just muscular. When you've heaved sacks of potatoes at 14, you get used to your body giving you gyp.'

Psychological issues

Some of the 'hidden' losses in this scenario are:

- a fatherless childhood
- poor material circumstances
- insensitive schooling
- two wives (although it is clear that the second wife was seen as something of a liability).

Could the lack of a father have made this character more inclined to proving himself as a manly man? He is conveyed as being 'working-class', a label which has less meaning than it used to. Yet his 'us/them' approach to healthcare and his reluctance to admit to pain support the traditional attitudes of the working-class man. (Men are three times less likely to seek advice for their health.[1]) His relationship to his body is that of master to servant. He expects it to operate in a functional way and he either has a high pain threshold or he has acquired a mindset which does not let it bother him.

His job was his identity. Whether he was heaving sacks of potatoes or looking after the school or mending people's cars, he needed to see himself as 'necessary'. Perhaps his deepest loss is this loss of being needed, which is probably why he insists on looking at the nurse's car. Being given the jigsaw, a well-meant gift is not perceived as therapeutic, we can infer. There is also more than a hint of isolation in his life as he misses the children from the school. We do not know whether he has had children but we understand that he has lived on his street for a long time. Is there a loss here of community spirit? It is a different challenge, doing a 2000-piece jigsaw with company rather than alone.

Communication seems to be awry. There is either too little when he is left on the dialysis machine or too much when the nurse visits and never stops talking. The ambulance driver encourages him to discuss the world's problems, which may serve to make him feel part of things, but the subject matter is generally more negative than positive. What might be the long-term effects of being called 'daft' for stammering at school? Is he less likely to ask questions about the kidney problems 'they' have identified?

There is the unfortunate fact that EBM (evidence-based medicine) is the acronym of the initials of his first wife. The confusion upsets him and he has a bit of incontinence, which leads to more anxiety about being put in sheltered accommodation. We get the impression of somebody trying to conceal problems from the professionals. The newspapers have informed him about life expectancy, which has encouraged him to adopt a fighting approach to survival, almost to beat the system?

Although we might like to think that we are moving away from the traditional class-ridden society, it is apparent in this scenario that 'class' in the sense of stratification is alive and well. Could it ever be otherwise, do you think? We do not create divisions based on family background or education so much now, but we are all caught up, to a greater or lesser degree in the competition for material wealth and status symbols. Perhaps this patient has hastened his end by the construction of the patio facilities for his second wife?

Personal and professional development

1 Reflect on the degree to which your job is your identity. If you wear a uniform, do you feel more secure in it than out of it? Does it give you pleasure to wear an identity badge? How far does work provide you with a sense of belonging?

2 If you were to lose your job, what feelings would you have? Looking back on your work history, think about the way the roles you performed changed your sense of yourself.

3 What sort of attitudes do you hold towards elderly patients? How do you think the system might be improved to preserve a sense of individuality and belonging to a rapidly changing society?

4 Reflect on your use of language with patients. If you consider the range of talking from light chat to the delivery of serious clinical information, where do you think your strengths and weaknesses lie?

5 We live in times where belief in 'the talking cure' prevails. The ambulance driver connects with the patient but the topic is the same one each time – the troubles in the world. How far does talking about negative things release feelings and how far do you think it reinforces negative attitudes?

6 Looking at your experience of training in healthcare, were there critical incidents which contributed to the development of the qualities of sensitivity or toughness?

7 What do you think of the exchange of car maintenance and jigsaw puzzles here?

8 In your professional career to date, do you think that you have succeeded in changing men's attitudes to their bodies? How?

9 What skills would you adopt with this patient to enable him to be more honest about his pain?

10 What are the advantages and disadvantages of this man living alone or in sheltered accommodation?

Useful tip
People remember the beginnings and endings of messages most easily. Check your communication skills and social skills for first and last impressions.

Reference

1 Sandman D *et al.* (2000) *Out of Touch: American men and the health care system.* The Commonwealth Fund, New York.

K is for Kids

'It's not like *Casualty* on the television. You don't get all these nurses having time to sort your life out. When I got the call from my ex-wife that our son, Mike had been rushed into hospital, I was in the middle of a big business deal in Paris. I hadn't been in to a hospital since my grandmother had died and so much of my life is spent in hotel rooms watching the television, I think I'd expected it to be more like *ER* than it was in the children's ward back in England.

When Mike was diagnosed with cystic fibrosis, it started the long process of the break-up between Karen and me. At first we said all the right things to each other, about how it was nobody's fault and that we would work together to make sure he had as normal a life as possible, but when she refused to try for another baby, I got restless. I don't mean I played away from home. I mean that if she didn't want another baby it meant that somehow she was really rejecting Mike, or rather the risk of another Mike. She always put it a different way. She said that she loved Mike so much she wasn't sure if she would have enough love left for another child. I really wanted a daughter. Everybody else has two children, so why should we miss out?

The children's ward was quiet when I got there. I was surprised at the colourful pictures on the walls. It brought a lump to my throat, the contrast between the toys and the deal I'd just secured for the company before catching the next flight to London. The staff were completely in control of the situation. So was my wife. She didn't acknowledge me when I got to the bedside. Mike was asleep but they had had to fight to keep him alive earlier in the day. I wanted the facts but the night nurse could only offer reassurance as she had just come on her shift. She looked very young. I had always felt touchy since the breakdown of the marriage because whoever does the moving out looks like they're doing the rejecting. But the fact is, I would have stayed on if Karen had let me. There was something about the dark quiet of the ward that made me want to confide in this nurse. I blurted out some things about not being the guilty party and she smiled. Karen appeared at the nurse's station and gave us both a bitter look. I said I'd go and spend the night at a hotel and come back in the morning.

The ward was different the next day. It seemed to be full of junior doctors in white coats and paediatricians in ordinary clothes. The nice nurse had gone and I was trying to work out who to speak to. It's strange. I am normally so confident in the business world but the sight and smell of so much illness almost paralysed me. A child was walking away from me attached to a drip on wheels and I did not know whether it was my son or not. Suddenly Karen appeared at my side. She told me that Mike was somewhere else in the hospital having some tests. She didn't look at me. She turned to go and added a muttered "thanks for turning up". I needed to know what was going on. She told me to ask the experts.

A senior nurse approached me. I started telling her who I was and asking her what was going on. She must have been on an assertiveness course because she politely persuaded me to wait five minutes as she had somebody else to attend to. I told her I'd got a special flight home to be with my boy. She was politely firm and explained that she had already promised the *mother* of another child that she would be available for a 'private word' and that she had to fulfil that obligation first.

I've never been a patient person. But I made myself sit down and count to 10. There was so much expertise walking around and yet nobody could tell me straightaway what was going on. I was furious about the tone she'd used with me. Then a male nurse came over and pulled up a chair and calmly explained the wider situation. They were in the middle of alterations to the ward and so everything was rushed that day. Mike, he told me, had just gone to the physiotherapist and would be back soon. He got me a drink, patted my shoulder and I started to relax.

Mike was fine in himself, though I could hardly believe how tall he'd grown. I'd bought him some chocolate animals at the airport. He hugged me but I had this feeling that he didn't want to be seen with his dad and children's chocolate.'

Psychological issues

The first issue here is the effect of the media's presentation of the health service. This man has not been in a hospital since his grandmother died and, after an emergency call and a flight, he finds himself in the quiet darkness of a children's ward. He experiences three different approaches from the nurses:

- the supportive smile from a young nurse
- the assertive approach from an older female nurse
- the time, drink and touch from a male nurse.

He and his wife are deeply estranged and the source of this problem is seen as the birth of Mike with the genetically inherited cystic fibrosis. Throughout the scenario the father feels defensive about his absence and angry about the emphasis on the word 'mother' by the older nurse. A busy businessman, he regrets the fact of his wife's unwillingness to have more children. What do you make of his thinking that everybody else has two children so why should he miss out?

The effect of different shifts on the ward is a factor in the additional struggles that the father experiences. Until the male nurse sits down with him, he does not realise why the ward is so full of experts (but little information) in the morning, because of the imminent building work. He says he wants facts more than reassurance, but by the end of the scenario it is the reassuring sight and hugs with his son that secure a sense of well-being.

Perceptions in acute care are almost invariably based on impressionistic evidence. There is little time to look beneath the surface. The father is gleaning what he can by the presence of white coats or ordinary clothes. Perhaps he appears at first sight to be a smartly dressed and successful man who has neglected his wife and son? He shows his impatience and has to wait. If we try and put ourselves in his shoes, or rather his mind, it could be a difficult shift for him to move from the values of the business deal in Paris to the tenderness of the children's ward.

Personal and professional development

1 How far do you think you were influenced in your choice of career by media images of the health service?
2 Reflect on working with divorced people – parents and children. Even though they may be a norm now in society regarding the 40–50% of marital or relationship breakdown, this does not reduce the pain of the individuals experiencing it. It may make people feel less unusual, but any loss of relationship carries the pain of thinking about 'what might have been', what went wrong, whose 'fault' was it, and so on. Emotions of rejection and (unhelpful) questions about blame may continue for years.
3 Reflect on your own experience of families and relationships. What feelings have you experienced around loss when these relationships have either changed or broken down? What helped you through?
4 Research the literature relating to cystic fibrosis. Consider the effects of having a child with a genetically inherited condition.
5 Facts and reassurance are necessary. Do you think that you get the balance right?
6 It is easy to become institutionalised yourself if you work in a hospital for a long time, not out of any unprofessional intent necessarily, but the

repetition of routines and the habits of care may limit our humanity. What do you think can be done to limit this?

7 Inconsistency of personal style (smiles/touches/assertiveness) may unsettle the stressed relative, if sufficient time isn't provided at the first encounter to assess clearly the needs of the visitor. Beginnings and endings of encounters are the bits that matter the most; they are what we remember. Does the team you work with maintain an awareness of this fact, do you think?

8 Perceptions can vary according to a multiplicity of factors:

- tiredness
- mood
- what you ate last night
- what you have to look forward to
- who a patient reminds you of
- whether a relative shows you respect.

Imagine a candle burning like a pilot light inside you. What is the flame like now? Is it tall and strong? Is it middling and jumpy? Is it almost out?

9 List the factors that you think make a good children's ward.

10 Loss of a child or children is probably the worst stress a human being can experience. Reflect on the *lack* of a child, as in this case, where the father wants to have a daughter too. What sort of emotions do you think men or women experience if their partner does not want a child or another child?

L is for Love

'When did I first feel depressed? Did I have a happy childhood? These are the questions I've been asked all my adult life. I have tried everything – from psychiatry to religion via homeopathy and massage. The first time I got really low, I was at university when I had just lost a friend and still hadn't managed to find a boyfriend. The psychiatrist said nothing for a year. His only contribution was: "There were a lot of power struggles in your family and the child in you comes out a lot".

It was hard to agree to see a psychiatrist in the first place, but at least he was at the health centre. The next person I tried was the student counsellor who inhabited a small Portakabin on the campus. She was a big woman who told me she loved me unconditionally. She had been trained in Rogerian techniques and never stopped smiling and nodding her head.

Then, in a different town in my early 20s, suffering another broken relationship and believing that it must be all my fault, that there must be something wrong with me, I sought the help of another psychiatrist. After a year, he said, sadly "Nobody deserves anything". Keen as ever to believe in the experts, I internalised this advice and tried to lower my expectations about life, love and the notion that youth is the best time of your life. On reflection, I think he was talking to himself. He had come out of Eastern Europe in difficult circumstances. He also asked me if I had fantasies about him being attracted to me.

And so it went on. Scared of being left on the shelf in my late 20s, I married a psychologist. He was cerebral and strange and made little timetables of how much time we could spend together. It was like being a rat in a cage. Deciding to end the marriage was the most adult decision I had ever made and I lost everything as a result – my home, my connections with my original family, my job, and very nearly my mind. Collapsed one day in the remains of the marital home, after drinking half a bottle of Southern Comfort, the village vicar took me in and made me take control of my life by divorcing my husband on the grounds of adultery. He then packed me off to the local psychiatric hospital where my first sight was a queue of shuffling patients lining up for the drugs. I stayed one night, refused to let them take any blood or tap my knees for reflexes and, on my way out the next day asked the only psychiatrist I could find "What's wrong with me?". She had never met me but held a file with my name on. She replied, hesitantly, "You have a personality disorder". I went in to the local town in a state of dread wondering what such a label meant. I was obviously beyond repair, and certainly beyond help. Then I saw a book entitled *Suddenly Single*, bought it and spent the rest of the day reading some reassuring advice that separation and divorce are like bereavement and that you have to go through a grieving process, which can be a rough ride.

Eventually I bought my own house but a series of rebound relationships and the presence of a male lodger, who was necessary to cover the mortgage, led to a further depression. I hoped for 'asylum' at the local hospital. There was little peace or sleep (noisy patients and snoring patients) and very little therapeutic input. The next thing I tried was the more alternative help – weekends on 'bodywork', encounter groups, primal scream workshops and eventually the internet. Then I found an excellent GP. Although she never understood depression, she always gave generously of her time, and supplied sick notes when necessary. The guilt that often goes with depression, and the attitude of society to 'mental' illness, often made me unable to ask for time off work, even though I had resorted to crying quietly in the office toilets for years. By chance I discovered that MIND, the mental health charity operated both a telephone support service and a small facility running relaxation groups in a Portakabin.

Then the menopause started. The mood swings got worse. My GP referred me to the community mental health team and I experienced the mixture of skills in a range of community psychiatric nurses (CPNs). The ones that visited my house travelled in pairs and asked the usual questions about childhood. When I went to the centre, just when I found a really helpful nurse, he took up another job and I was back to my own resources. That's when I embarked on private psychotherapy at enormous cost. Over a period of 18 months I spent nearly £2000. At one point, I lost the power of speech at his surgery and had to drive home, over 50 miles in a state of mental disintegration. That state lasted for seven days and seven nights. The hell was the uncertainty about whether or not it would end. A good friend helped me to pay the bill. In retrospect I would not have paid him anything. I considered legal action, years later, but what grounds does a person have, if *under* a psychiatrist?'

Psychological issues

This woman is writing from the perspective of looking back on the effects of seeking help through the mental health services. It is unlikely that, in the presence of depression itself, she would have been able to stand back and evaluate the impoverished input. She has tried everything:

- psychiatry
- counselling
- psychotherapy
- 'bodywork weekends'
- CPNs
- marriage to a psychologist.

The menopause arrives, her suffering is intensified and we are left wondering what her future holds.

The medical model is limited by its thinking along the lines of diagnosis or treatment. She is tired of the same old questions:

- When did it start?
- Did you have a happy childhood?

These are the questions that try and assess the frequency, intensity and duration of the symptoms of depression so that the professional can get a picture of the condition. But is this the best way to approach somebody suffering from this complex condition? Being questioned can put people on the defensive. Depression always has an eternal quality to it, so asking how long it has been there is, in fact, very depressing. The questions about child-hood reflect the professional's training bias towards believing that emotional problems stem from the first five years of life. It seems strange to ask this, because children between birth and five do not have the cognitive develop-ment to use language like adults and so the adult being questioned is, at best, cobbling together some mixture of memories which may or may not repre-ent the reality she or he experienced in those early years.

The psychiatric hospitals do not provide asylum – noise, lack of sleep, drug queues, diagnoses given in passing. She finds out, *by chance*, that MIND runs a helpline and a relaxation centre. Her GP is described as excellent both for her willingness to try and understand the condition (which means a generous investment of time) and her practical contribution with sick notes. We can equally imagine that, *by chance*, she might not have had such a GP. The CPNs are perceived as 'travelling in pairs' and the one who is very help-ful moves on to another job.

The patient, in pain and frustration, and yet still searching for the elusive professional help now pays £2000 to a private therapist who reduces her to a state of loss of speech.[1]

This scenario is entitled 'loss of love', and we read about a series of broken relationships. She finds a book that explains that divorce is hard work emotionally. There is some support from this text and a certain placing of her pain within the 'normal' range of human experience. To be reminded of a sense of belonging to normality can be an antidote to the painful stigma which still goes with depression.[2]

Personal and professional development

1 Think of the term 'depression'. Does it matter what words we use to name and to label things? What's the psychological difference between naming and labelling?
2 Reflect on your experience of low mood. Do you think you have had 'clinical depression'? What do you do to make yourself feel better if you are low? Can you apply your insights to your patients?
3 Loss reactions can be crudely configured into 'soft' and 'hard' aspects, crying being an example of the softness of sorrow and anger being an example of the harder side of the grieving process. Which emotions are you more comfortable with and what do you think this might say about you?
4 Reflect on your training and experience in 'mental' health. What do you think you learnt that was useful, what do you need to unlearn and what do you think you need to know now?
5 The questions we ask of our patients say a lot about ourselves (and our theoretical biases), but the patients may be less aware of this because they are feeling vulnerable at the time. Reflect on the use of questions in interviews with patients.
6 Imagine you control (some) NHS resources. How would you begin to rectify the problems in psychiatric facilities?
7 Imagine you are a nurse in a psychiatric ward. Think of a simple solution to the problem of snorers and non-snorers being placed next to each other.
8 What are your views about the role of CAM (complementary and alternative medicine) in depression?
9 Charities such as MIND can be sidelined. What might be done practically to stop this?
10 Research the literature to assess the EBM (evidence-based medicine) which supports or otherwise the prescribing of antidepressants by GPs.

Useful tip: When you're low, others (seem to) glow
Depression is so depressing that it distorts perceptions. Even if you cannot change your perceptions, telling yourself: 'I am depressed and that is why I see things negatively' may help you to separate the depression a little bit away from yourself. Then, you may feel a little less isolated or inferior to other people who *seem* to be getting on with life and/or enjoying it.

Useful tip

If you are feeling depressed, your mind defaults to a negative view very quickly – negative automatic thoughts (NATs). You need to swat these gnats with all your might. Or think of them as ANTs, tiny insects to be treated with the contempt they deserve. Try to distract yourself as suggested in Butler and Hope's *Manage Your Mind* (*see* Further reading).

References

1 *Understanding Talking Treatments* (undated) MIND publications, London.

2 Anonymous author (2003) The highway from hell. *The Guardian Weekend*, 8 November.

M is for Memory

'Looking back now, I can see that it began a long time ago. At the time, I couldn't understand what was wrong. I thought there was something wrong with me. Dennis was so cross all the time, so critical. Everything I did seemed to be wrong, and everyone else was in the wrong. In fact, at one time, Dennis actually suggested I should leave. He became very moody. Of course, now, I can see that most of the time he was covering up. I remember the day I knew for certain that something was seriously wrong. I was tidying in his room and I found a whole drawer full of bills. They went back months ... and all unpaid. Dennis had always taken care of the money. I sat down with him and he cried ... said he didn't know what to do anymore. That's when we made an appointment to see the doctor. Well, by the time we went in, he was fine again. The doctor asked him how he was and he said "fine". So I had to say "No he isn't.". I said that his memory was very bad. Dennis was furious with me, and the doctor wasn't much good. He said that it was 'just old age' and that there was nothing that could be done. I went home and cried. In the end, it was the district nurse who encouraged me to go back and ask to be referred to the specialist. That was another horrible time. We went to see this man and he asked Dennis all these questions. Of course, Dennis looked to me to help him but I was told I couldn't so I had to just sit there. Dennis blamed me for putting him through that. The specialist said that Dennis had Alzheimer's. In a way, it was a relief. It wasn't me. There was something seriously wrong.

The family has all been very supportive. Of course, Philip our eldest lives a long way away so he can't come up all that often. His work takes up a lot of his time. Janet, our daughter comes and helps as often as she can, but she has her own family to look after. I try not to bother her. Mostly we manage on our own. Dennis goes to a day centre now. He needs help with everything. It's hard for both of us. He was always the one in charge and now I have to tell him what to do. He was a manager and put everything into his work. Now he spends a lot of his time wandering from room to room. He can't stay still. It drives me mad. He has no conversation. We used to discuss everything and now we can't talk about anything. Lately I find I keep crying for no reason. I get very tired. Of course, the nights are disturbed. I'm always half listening in case Dennis gets up. He doesn't know where the bathroom is and I'm worried that he might fall down the stairs. The family all think I need a break. They are trying to arrange respite care but it's not that easy. I don't think I could relax with Dennis somewhere else. They wouldn't know how to look after him like I do. Dennis would hate it. He's never been a mixer. And those places are full of old people.

Our friends are getting older. Tim and Anne were our closest friends but Anne died three years ago and Tim isn't well. He's had a stroke and can't get out. We always used to go and see them but that was when Dennis was able to drive. I never learnt; I never needed to. That's the trouble with getting older. A lot of our friends have died and those that are alive, they're not so mobile. Some people seem to have just stayed away since Dennis became ill. I think the illness scares them. To be honest, I tend to avoid seeing people now. I'm never quite sure what Dennis is going to do and I don't want him embarrassed. Mealtimes are difficult. He makes a terrible mess. I know it's not his fault but he used to be so smart and now he doesn't seem to care.

Sometimes I feel very alone. There's no one to talk to. I don't know how I'm going to carry on. But I have to. Dennis and I have been together for nearly 60 years. We always promised to look after each other 'in sickness and in health'. I can't abandon him now. I don't know what I would do without him. Sometimes we sit there and the old Dennis says something. He was always very witty. Well, I just have to soldier on.'

Psychological issues

The key psychological issue here is that the carer is suffering as much as the patient. How could it be otherwise? When people have been married for nearly 60 years, their separate identities are likely to be blurred. The marriage is a traditional one, in the sense that Dennis did the 'manly' things and his wife did the caring things. She suffers particularly in the appointment with the specialist when she is coerced into not covering up for her husband.

There is also evidence that Dennis has been 'in denial'. Observing somebody effectively saying that s/he does not believe that s/he is ill, can engage us in irritation and even confrontation.

We can also glean that Dennis's wife is 'in denial' in a more subtle way, in that she first describes the family as being 'very supportive' but then goes on to describe a busy son and a daughter preoccupied with her own family.

There is the fact, too, of the disease being variable and inconsistent. Towards the end of the scenario, we realise that parts of the original Dennis occasionally shine through. His wit, for example, can sometimes come alive. But this may add an extra poignancy to the wife's loss, as it serves as a reminder of how things used to be. Mixed losses are sometimes called 'ambiguous loss'. Perhaps all loss is, strictly speaking, ambiguous. We are not in the land of light and dark but shades of grey. Things are not always as black and white as we might wish them to be, simply for the sake of clarity.

The doctor makes not just the wrong diagnosis but no diagnosis. Telling somebody that 'it is just old age' could be construed as evidence for the lack of time given to GPs under the NHS. Equally, it could demonstrate a lack of diagnostic ability, or insensitivity or impatience. The doctor is faced with conflicting descriptions – the wife saying the husband's memory is very bad, the husband saying that he is fine. However, there is a risk that elderly people are increasingly marginalised. The fact that the term 'rationalisation' of resources has crept into discussions about the future of the NHS cannot but frighten older people that they may be the first to lose out. Why? Because we live in a capitalist economy, which tends to place first value on those who are the most viable economic units, that is, the young.

The specialist hurts the wife. By placing her in the same room as her husband while he undergoes the tests, but by insisting that she does not help (for justifiable scientific reasons/the need for rigorous results), he unwittingly creates marital tension. Could this be done differently? Yes. The wife could be invited to sit or talk with a caring member of staff while her husband is 'tested'. That is, if multidisciplinary teams were more of a reality than a rhetoric.

The district nurse is the clinical key in the chain of events in this scenario.

Labelling plays a part. The wife is almost relieved to be told that Dennis has Alzheimer's. How strange is the human mind! How we dislike uncertainty. Once she has the label to which she can pin the behaviours of her husband, she knows what she is facing, however bad that news might be. As mentioned previously in this book, it is important to make the subtle distinction between naming and labelling. Naming clarifies; labelling stigmatises.

He's demented.   He's got dementia.   It's Alzheimer's.

The first is pejorative, the second victimises and the third is objective but cold.

Personal and professional development

1 Reflect on your experience of caring for the elderly. The elderly may be as vulnerable as babies, but they may not look as appealing! They may not be able to voice their concerns and they may not have a wife, husband, daughter, son or friend to advocate on their behalf. How comfortable are you in the role of advocate?

2 Put yourself in the shoes of the GP in this scenario, when he finds out later that he has missed the diagnosis. Do you think that training courses are the best way to update healthcare professionals? Think of the amount

of time it takes for a morning, afternoon or day out of the clinical area. Think of the evidence which suggests that we may forget quite quickly what we have learnt in a one-off training session. Could the technology be used better? Could there be 'reminders' sent to primary care, from, for example the BMA (British Medical Association), about things such as misdiagnosis? What would be the advantages and disadvantages of such a plan?

3 Reflect on your experience of multidisciplinary teams. What have been the best and worst clinical outcomes of:

- working alone
- working in a team?

4 Have you worked with patients and carers where Alzheimer's and other forms of dementia have played a part? In this scenario, it could be argued that the wife is suffering more loss than the husband, in the sense that she is well enough to perceive clearly. Holistic medicine, therefore, in this case, is double the work: there are two patients in effect.

5 Reflect on marriages or partnerships that you know well. Is dependency an inevitable feature?

6 Reflect on your own feelings about growing older. The ageing process starts, biologically, at about 25 years of age. Many people (particularly women) express anxiety about reaching 30 years of age. And yet we are living longer and longer. What does this say about ageism and sexism in our society?

7 The specialist in this scenario could have been more sensitive. Is there a sense in which the hierarchical structures of the NHS encourage people to become arrogant, as they climb the ladder to 'success'? Why do some people still believe that consultants are more important than nurses? If you were to redesign the NHS, what sort of structure would you choose?

8 How would you help this couple if you were their community nurse? Prioritise a plan.

9 Evaluate the advantages and disadvantages of being told you have dementia or Alzheimer's. Think of access to drugs too.

10 Tearfulness and loneliness are affecting the wife. What prevents GPs from liaising with charities such as the Alzheimer's Society early on in the process of the illness?

Useful tip
The website www.memoryclinic.com is a good place to start if you or someone you know has any worries about memory loss.

Useful address
Alzheimer's Society
Gordon House
10 Greencoat Place
London SW1P 1PH

Alzheimer's Helpline 0845 300 0336

N is for Nurse

'I was only 29 years old when I found the lump. It was when I was pregnant, so no sooner had I come out of hospital with Jake then I had to go back in for it to be removed from my breast.

That was five years ago and I have been struggling the whole time with cancer. Poor Jake has never really had a mother and he is now suffering panic attacks at school. My husband has just been promoted at work when really he wants to be at home with me. I never actually say to myself that I am dying, but nor do I deny the fact that it is very likely. I am lucky. I have a strong religious faith. If it is God's will that I do not see my son reach his sixth birthday, then I can accept that. My husband is less accepting. Is it harder to watch somebody you love suffer, than to suffer yourself?

The last bout of chemotherapy made me feel as if my body was on fire from head to toe. The last tests at the hospital showed that my liver has 'secondaries'. It is swollen and I cannot eat very well because I'm just sick.

My mother has managed to fly over from Baghdad. It has not been easy for her. The political situation means that she has trouble getting out. When you are as ill as I am, you cannot believe that bureaucracy and politics can be like they are.

The Macmillan nurse, Susie, has been visiting every day. She is wonderful. She is also very good with my mother and Jake, who need as much care as I do. Mick and I discussed things after the last trip to hospital. We decided that we did not want me to go in to a hospice. I lie in bed all day and when Jake comes home from school, we hold each other on the bed. Then Susie makes everyone a drink, my mum plays with Jake downstairs and Mick arrives home from work early to hold my hand. He can't stop crying. I am letting go and he is holding on.

Susie and I have only known each other a few weeks and yet it is as if we have always been friends. She is younger than I am and yet she is so mature — gentle and strong. I have tried to tell her that I know I am going home to God but I sense that she does not have the sort of faith that I have. I am trying to convince her so that she can persuade Mick that everything will be all right after I am gone. I am worried that Mick is a bit envious of her and the way we can talk about everything.

I am getting weaker all the time. It is hard. I wake up sometimes and I am not sure that I am still here. My mother-in-law who rings up every day sounds very far away on the phone. She is coming to stay. That will really help Mick and Jake, I hope.

Today is sad. Susie cannot visit. She rang to say that she has a very bad cold and does not want to risk infecting me. They are sending Steve instead. I want to say that I don't care if she infects me. I want to tell her how much I like her. I cannot tell her that I feel that I do not have much time left. I know that she is one of those nurses who could never say 'no' to me or anyone in need. I know that she thinks she is doing the best. Mick senses that I really want her and says that he will make a fuss if I like. He has changed a lot since my illness. He never used to stand up for himself. It is strange, dying. I can see so clearly.

Steve is not like Susie. He is good at his job. But he is not Susie.'

Psychological issues

The psychological issue here is the effect on the mind of finding a lump and discovering that it is cancer. What must this be like? Invasion? Betrayal? The fact that healthcare professionals have such difficulty telling patients that they have cancer indicates the level of dread associated with this disease.[1] We even refer to it as the C-word, whereas heart disease and strokes are not translated into the H- and S-words, respectively. No matter how much research and publicity is presented to us about the progress in conquering this disease, it still holds a mysterious power, a terror. The sense of a loss of control over the body, the body with which we have been familiar (and maybe even taken for granted) since birth, is horrific; the imagination may take over, picturing the cells reproducing themselves and spreading to infinity.

The timing of this woman's disease could not be worse – just before the birth of her baby. Life and death, hand-in-hand, and the place of the lump, her breast at such a young age is tragic. She describes herself as being lucky in that she has a strong religious faith. She believes that death is not the end. She is hoping that she will 'go home' to God.

Jake, Mick and her mother are suffering. They cannot let go. Jake is only five and he is understandably traumatised, not just by the imminent loss of his mother but by the lack of her presence since birth. This is a family in crisis. If this were not enough, her mother has had difficulty coming over from Baghdad due to the continuing Iraqi war.

In spite of the seeming difference in religious outlook, the patient and Susie have formed a deeply communicative relationship. The patient is concerned that her husband is feeling left out and even envious. She is glad that his mother is coming to visit to support him and Jake.

Then we have the 'last straw' event of Susie deciding not to visit for fear of infecting the patient. Steve is competent but the quality of relationship is not there. Mick, who has grown a lot through his wife's illness, is going to make a fuss and try and get the other nurse back. The patient senses that her death is near and yet does not want to make a fuss or be demanding. 'Contrary to popular belief ... dying people know they are dying ... '.[2]

Personal and professional development

1 Reflect on your experience with cancer, either in your personal life or your professional life.
2 What sort of evidence is there for patients like this, who are very mild-mannered being more prone to getting breast cancer?
3 Do you agree with the Macmillan nurse's decision not to visit? How comfortable are you with saying 'no', in your personal life and in your professional life?
4 Put yourself in Steve's shoes. What do you think his priorities should be?
5 Do you have a particular religious faith? How comfortable are you talking to patients and relatives about death and dying?
6 Giving bad news (*see* B for Baby) can be very difficult. Write out a script for yourself detailing how you would tell each of these people – the mother in Baghdad, Mick, Jake, Mick's mother. If you were to phone the mother, would you consider leaving the message on an answer phone?
7 What are the disadvantages of phrases like 'passing over', 'gone to sleep', 'gone home to Jesus'?
8 Assuming the patient is right in her judgement that she has very little time left, how would you help Jake, Mick and her mother after she has died?
9 Do you agree with the family's decision for Jake to continue going to school, even though he is suffering panic attacks?
10 What are the advantages and disadvantages of dying in a hospice or at home?

References

1 Groopman J (2002) Dying words: How should doctors deliver bad news? *The New Yorker.* 28th October.

2 Callanan M and Kelley P (1992) *Final Gifts.* Hodder & Stoughton, London.

O is for Opportunities

'I love hospital. I'm what they call a 'regular'. The nurses and I have a laugh and the last time I was in the hydrotherapy pool, one of them threatened to drown me, saying it was the only way they'd ever get me to die!

I was the victim of a massive RTA (road traffic accident) five years ago. I was 25 years old then and had my own business. I was driving home when I was hit by a car. It took them four hours to cut me out of the wreckage. I'd broken my neck, ruptured my spleen, shattered my face, smashed my frontal lobes, torn my arm and lost my foot. But I'm fine today. I was in a coma for two and a half months, in a wheelchair for two years and the consultant said that I'd never walk or talk again. I proved him wrong. My mum's beaten cancer and my sister's had a triple by-pass. They said my sister's heart trouble was because of all the worry she had, looking after my mum and me, but I just laughed.

I can be cheerful now but it wasn't always like that. I lost my girlfriend. She said: "I don't want to be with a cripple". I lost my lifestyle; I had travelled the world before my accident and made a lot of money. My family said that when I was in the ICU I had hallucinated that I had been dealing on the stock market. I really believed these things. It must have been the drugs. I lost my sense of future. That's been the toughest. I'm not too sure who I am now. I still look snazzy. The compensation from the accident has made sure of that. The QC made sure that I could get a butler from London to look after me so that I could keep my independence. But he didn't do things the way I wanted them done. I asked him to make me a tuna sandwich one day. I managed to get my wheelchair into the kitchen and I saw him squeezing out the tuna from the tin with his bare hands. I was angry. I had had a serious infection in hospital and the last thing I needed was more germs. He replied "Father worked at the Savoy. And that is how they squeezed tuna there. And that is how I intend to carry on squeezing tuna". I sacked him on the spot.

I spend a lot of time with my sister. She drives me around, helps me to get out of the house and that. I'm still not quite right. I'm having to wear a bag and they think I'm going to be impotent forever. That's the next thing I want to prove wrong. But will a girlfriend ever fancy me? I'm covered in scars and I'm blind in one eye and there's a bolt through my neck to hold my head on. The nurse said that if I shake my head too hard, it might fall off. You see what

I mean? They're a great laugh. My sister and I try and keep a lot from our mum. She was told she would not live for more than a few months, and that was 10 years ago. "Mind over matter", that's what we all say.

Sometimes we get cross when we hear people moan about colds and tooth-ache. We want to convince other people to make the most of their health while they've got it. I could never have guessed that I would have been in that car accident five years ago.

Last week, I asked one of the nurses for a date. She's a student on the ward so there shouldn't be a problem. I'm really excited about my next visit because I'm confident she is going to say "yes", even though she did say that she would think about it and get back to me. She is just like the girlfriend I lost, she even has the same name. I think my luck is about to change.'

Psychological issues

The first impression is that this patient is institutionalised. It is rare to hear such enthusiastic expressions of joy about being in hospital. As we read on, we could infer that one reason why he is so cheerful is because he has survived such a serious accident. Is he too cheerful?

Although the patient conveys that he is enjoying the humour of the nurses, we might want to be a bit careful about believing that all patients would enjoy being told that the only way to make them die is to drown them in the hydrotherapy pool. Being told not to shake your head in case it falls off, is another example of humour which might misfire with somebody feeling vulnerable.

The prediction that he will not walk or talk, has been unproven. How appropriate is it for medical staff to make predictions, either about prognoses or the expected time of a person's death?

We get the impression that this patient is part of a determined family all of whom have had serious health problems. They say that they have adopted the 'mind over matter' approach to their advantage. Is there any suggestion that there might be 'denial' operating here?

Some of the extra losses mentioned are:

- the loss of a girlfriend
- loss of a lifestyle
- loss of future plans
- loss of identity.

He reassures himself that he still looks 'snazzy'. Perhaps his image conscious-ness is a reflection of his age?

He is looking forward to the response from the student nurse. What do you make of the fact that he is also attracted to her because she has the same name as his former girlfriend? Optimistic to the end, we might fear for him being disappointed. In between optimism and pessimism is realism, a hard balancing point. We could argue that we live in rather cynical times and at least he's not a cynic!

Television programmes about medicine, such as *Casualty* and *ER* often focus on the romantic relationships between the characters. How do you think members of staff might best handle invitations to date? Is this where the humour of banter comes in? Pretending not to take it seriously?

Personal and professional development

1 Reflect on your use of humour with colleagues and patients. Medical humour, partly due to the effects of the training (e.g. the need to distance yourself from some of the gory aspects) can be perceived as quite earthy and tough. Practitioners may need to be able to laugh amongst themselves about orifices and hairy parts.

2 Re: doctors' prognoses? Here's a riddle: What's the difference between God and doctors? (Answer: God knows He's not a doctor.)

3 'They said that my sister's heart trouble was due to all the worry looking after me.' How often do you think that things are said that may be overheard by patients?

4 He may have hallucinated in the ICU. Research the literature on 'ICU syndrome'.

5 Reflect on your experience of clinical boundaries and the temptation to blur them.

6 Do you think the effect of this accident (including the blindness in one eye and the body scars) would be different for a woman? What does this say about sexism in society?

7 We are habituated to hearing about small to large sums paid in compensation for accidents. If you were a policy maker, would you change this? Are there other ways of compensating people apart from money? What do you think of moves towards the American system of potentially greater litigation in the health service?

8 How would you counsel this man towards a new future?

9 The Freudian defence mechanism, denial, would seem to be a successful means of cutting out pain for the individual. But it comes at a cost, a cost to the individual and to those around him. The individual has to work to block out negative realities and because this is a path away from the truth,

it will always be a hiding to nothing. The people around the individual suffer from frustration if they can see through the denial and they may, in a spirit of love, try to break through the barrier, only to find themselves on the receiving end of anger. The anger is a mask for the fear, fear of the truth, fear of the whole story with all its elements, good and bad. Reflect on your use of this defence mechanism.

10 The Freudian defence mechanism 'reaction formation' could be applied to this patient. Does his happiness seem to be a bit hollow? Freud might have argued that the dynamic swing to the polar opposite of the pain (of loss, here) to a resounding joy, is a defence mechanism used unconsciously to protect the core of the person from anxiety. Assuming that you can access your 'unconscious', reflect on your use of this defence. The simplest way to think about this is to reflect on the times when you have felt driven to put a brave face on things. You might have walked around with a fixed smile. Supposing you have been let down by a friend. You run into them out of the blue. Instead of frowning or glaring, you put on a big smile.

Useful tip
The sense of loss of opportunity might be a hidden loss in many situations because we live in a competitive society and illness holds us back.

P is for Power

'I think I've got pre-natal depression. I've got morning sickness too. It's my fifth baby and the other four are a bit of a handful. There's Ryan, he's 16 and just got his babe pregnant (and I'd bought him 100 condoms for his birthday). Then there's Brooklyn and she's 14 and her period is late. Then there's Annabelle and she's three and won't come out of nappies. And then there's Angel-Rose and she's one and still wanting breastfeeding.

Clint has had to give up work. He'd had a pop round, delivering pop from the back of his van, but there's been some sort of trouble with the pop people. They couldn't get their deliveries to him on time and he'd made these promises on the estate. He'd done these special offers for parties and it's all gone wrong.

I look after myself. I get the catalogues and I'm always ordering the latest. The health visitor says I should be giving the family five fruit and vegetables a day. She says they should have these different colours, red, yellow and green. They get them on their pizzas and we all have ketchup on our chips. The social worker (he's cute) says that they'll take the kids off me if I don't get myself together. He said I was 'vulnerable' but they have these courses. I told him I want to be a midwife. He said I'd have to train as a nurse first. I said "I already am one." (Angel had just bumped her head and I was sticking a plaster on it). He said "Are you being realistic?" I said "I'm as real as this fag". He said "You should give up smoking when you're pregnant." I told him where to go. He went. I got a letter from the SS (social services). They said they could take Angel off me for bruises and bumps. I'd kill them if they tried.

I never wanted a big family. But it just took off. I had Ryan when I was 17 years old. They wrote about me on my notes in the hospital: 'Young mother/watch'. Then Brooklyn was an accident. Then Annabelle was after I got raped after a karaoke night at the Working Men's Club. And I had to have Angel to teach them a lesson at the hospital. They'd written about me again. It was after Annabelle was born. The delivery was like I'd had to push out a truckload of pop cans. The bloke in the suit had written on that card at the end of my bed 'mandatory sterilisation'. Clint kicked up a fuss when he saw it. He told them where to put their mandatory.

I've got these pains but I think it's just the baby growing inside me. I don't like doctors. Clint says I should go to the antenatal. But the other mums look at me like I'm daft. We're having problems with the Housing at the council offices. They keep threatening to kick us out. The electric's been disconnected but Clint's mum's new partner gave us a gas cooker and fitted it for free. It was my birthday at the weekend and Clint got me a little dog from the rescue place. He's cool. He's not house-trained yet so we've got him on a chain in the back yard. Trouble is, he's got a bit of a bark on him and the neighbours have started to complain.

The pains have been getting worse. The health visitor told me I had to go for a check-up. It turns out that I've got a baby stuck in my tubes. 'Ectopic pregnancy' they wrote in my notes. They also had a good look round inside and I've got all these bits that are in the wrong place. So it looks like I'll be sterile anyway. I can't stop crying. I love babies. You forget that they change and then end up as teenagers. We've just been fined for not having a TV licence. I couldn't live without my TV. It's company when Clint's out with his mates. I saw this programme about the richest people in Britain. I'm going to have my hair done like one of them.

I can't believe it! Clint's just come back from his mum's. They've won the jackpot on the lottery and they're going to share it with us. All our problems are over. We're going to move to the States and have a condominium with its own pool.'

Psychological issues

The circumstances in which this woman initially finds herself could be described as those of the 'underclass' in Great Britain. She and her family have a poor diet and poor housing. They are marginalised to the point of being flung to the edges of the system, whether that system is the state, or the social or health services of the state.

She sees looking after herself as buying things from the catalogues but she is smoking while pregnant. Pizzas, pop, chips and ketchup are a large part of her family's diet. We get the impression that the dietary advice from the health visitor has been misunderstood. The social worker does not appear to have any authority in the face-to-face situation. But the SS are threatening her with the removal of her daughter.

She is angry with the hospital for writing things about her that are intrusive and pejorative. She is angry with the system and its representatives. She is depressed by the loss of her pregnancy and the demands of all the other members of the family.

She is a picture of powerlessness. If you can empathise with her and then compare her circumstance with, say, a minister in the government or a

Londoner with a private income, you might wonder how she has had the strength to continue. That is one perspective, a compassionate one. If she is seen through other eyes (or a neighbour subjected to the howls of the new dog!), her life might be construed as a 'sponger' off the welfare state.

She believes that the solution to all her problems is going to be sharing in the lottery win and moving across the Atlantic. She is already identifying with the rich by planning to have her hair done like somebody she has seen on the television.

Social class has changed dramatically in the last 50 years. Britain has always been known as a class-ridden (if not riddled) society. In previous centuries, class was ascribed according to ownership of land and family background. In the first half of the twentieth century, class began to be defined more as a result of education, thanks to the 'education for all' Education Act in 1870. But since the 1980s, people's positions in society have been greatly determined by the power of the cash they can access. The means by which the cash is acquired has become of less interest since the business boom of the Thatcherite years (1979–1997).

Personal and professional development

1 Reflect on your perception of the class to which you think you belong. We live in aspirational times. Do you feel driven to 'climb the ladder'? Where do you think you are going? Re-read the Introduction to this book. Are you focusing your life on 'having' at the expense of 'being'? Do you find yourself caught up in 'doing' with insufficient time to relax, to 'be'?

2 When have you experienced feelings of powerlessness? What were the consequences of these feelings and what did you do to alleviate them?

3 Have you worked in gynaecology, obstetrics, midwifery or infertility? How do these areas affect patients' sense of power?

4 Power is powerful. It adds to a sense of confidence and self-worth. Too much power can lead to arrogance. Too little power can lead to depression. Power is notoriously easy to abuse. Reflect on your observations on the uses and abuses of power in the microcosm of the clinical encounter and in the macrocosm of the health service.

5 Power, like beauty, is, to some degree, in the eye of the beholder. That is, it is a relative concept. That is why we say things like, 'Don't give them the power' or 'Don't let them get to you'. Do you think that the powerful should relinquish some power in favour of the powerless? How likely is this?

6 Imagine you are the health visitor working with this family before they won the lottery. Think of better ways to help them towards an improved diet.

7 Reflect on the use of written material in the health service – from patients' notes as in this case, to letters about appointments and test results. How could this important area be improved?

8 Think of the range of mixed feelings in a woman's mind during the nine months from conception to birth. Do antenatal clinics offer sufficient emotional support at this time in a woman's life?

9 The gap between rich and poor has grown increasingly wide since the 1980s. We also live in a culture that tends to name and shame (and to blame) through some parts of the press and media. Be honest with yourself. Do you have any thoughts or feelings of criticism towards this mother. If so, why? If not, why?

10 To what extent is money a solution to depression?

Q is for Questions

'I come to this UK from Poland. My English is not so good, and my wife, she has no English at all. We are starting to feel happy and our neighbours are all very welcoming and Katya is in the first year of high school when she is suddenly very ill. She come home one day with headache and sore throat. We always said we would not spoil our children so we tell her just to lie down for a while. Next thing, she is very hot and with convulsion. We panic. We do not know the system. The neighbours ring for the ambulance and very quickly she is admitted to the children's ward. We do not want to make a fuss, the staff are so busy but we want to know what is happening. I go ask to see the doctor. The nurse, he is very quick, and I do not understand a word he says but I trust him. I can tell he knows what he is doing just by his eyes, his smile and the way he touches my wife's arm. But I want a doctor. I want the answers: Is Katya going to die? What is wrong with her? Do we have to pay money? Can my wife get help too from this hospital? She has been ill too and I tell her it is just because she's getting used to this new country. In my country you go straight to hospital if you are only a little bit ill. We do not have what you call the 'primary care', the 'surgery'.

Then we see a man in a suit. He must be the one with the answers. I go to speak. He does not see me. I go to find the man-nurse. He is gone from his shift, they say. A lady who says she 'runs the ward' asks if she can help us. I explain we are foreign. She says they have interpreters for ethnic minorities like us and she will ring for one. She draws me a picture of Katya in bed in a special part of the hospital. She has 'infections'. They will make her better. They have drugs. We must wait and see. They will tell us when we can see her. She speaks so loudly she is shouting and she says it is because I am foreign. Is she assuming that I am deaf or stupid?

My wife, now, she is crying. Another kind person comes with tea trolley. She does not have a uniform. We do not know who she is. We want to ask her lots of things. She is not rushing. She has time. She sits with us. She is called 'Volunteer'. We tell her everything in our broken English. We do not care that she says nothing but it is the listening she gives us to our story. Then the interpreter arrives. He explains everything and tells us that Katya will be all right and that we must go home and rest, and that the hospital will take care of things. My wife wants to see her daughter very much but she is so distressed that we all decide that it is best if she does not.

Late that night, the neighbours come to say the hospital has telephoned for us to go straight there. We are scared. We think Katya is dying. She is very ill. She may not survive the night. My wife and I sit helplessly watching her fight for her life inside this big bubble thing. We are there for days. We pray very hard. I ask myself: "Was I right to leave my homeland?" "Is it the cold that has made her ill?" "Why am I not rich enough to have flat with the central heating?" "Will my wife survive the stress?" "Do I have a right to ask the hospital to check her heart?" "Should we ask for the priest?" I am as squeezed as a lemon with worry.

We are very relieved now. Katya came through it all 'with flying colours' the doctors said. My wife and I think that we will give the staff a special thank you. We are going to cook our national dish and take it in to the ward. Perhaps other children and their families will want to try my wife's cooking. There is no question about this one; her food is the best in the world.'

Psychological issues

Having undeveloped English, while your only daughter is seriously ill and your wife is suffering from stress, adds to the difficulties experienced by the father. Members of staff speak either too quickly or too loudly for him to be treated with the respect he deserves. Being new to any country makes a person more vulnerable and it is clear that this father takes his family responsibilities very seriously. He has many questions but he is frustrated.

The system is unhelpful to him at this point. He wants to see a doctor for a diagnosis. He thinks he sees a consultant (the man in the suit?) but whoever it is does not see him. He searches for the male nurse but he has left his shift and the woman who 'runs the ward' refers to him as an 'ethnic minority'. She upsets him with her insensitive way of communicating loudly. He and his wife find that they are given time and listening by the volunteer with the tea trolley.

Then the interpreter arrives, clears up the medical details but tells these adults what to do – to go home, rest and to leave everything to the hospital. The man's wife wants to see her daughter but he decides that she is too distressed.

Then they are called out in the night. They find themselves sitting outside a 'big bubble thing', watching helplessly as their daughter struggles with 'infections'. More questions come to his mind but these are private ones and he suffers their unanswerable quality on his own.

The child survives 'with flying colours'. They decide to make a special meal for the ward staff as thanks.

It is all too easy to make assumptions about people, particularly patients and relatives when relying on impressionistic evidence. 'First impressions are lasting impressions', we are told. For the father, the nurse in charge speaks too loudly as if assuming that he is deaf or stupid.

Useful tip
A useful adage is: **Do not assume**, i.e. Do not make an **ass** out of you and **me**.

Personal and professional development

1 Reflect on your experience of travel. Have you found yourself with inadequate language in difficult circumstances? Have you ever been ill abroad? In what ways did the different situation make you feel more vulnerable?

2 Think about times (perhaps at school/college/in your first healthcare placement) when you have had questions that you have not felt able or confident to express? What was the psychological effect of this?

3 Questions can put people on the defensive. Why? Is it partly because we have all been conditioned through 14 years of schooling to find an answer to a question, often in the public arena of the classroom where mistakes might be mocked? The 'Why do you do this?' question is one of the ones to avoid in the clinical area, particularly mental health, because it is demanding reasons for behaviour, reasons which patients may not have or be able to articulate.

4 The loss of the ability to question, particularly when you are a carer, watching the child you love suffer, is extremely stressful. How could the staff have communicated better?

5 The system of communication is what has broken down in this example. We have the ward manager, the male nurse, the interpreter and the volunteer. Reflect on your experience of good and bad teams in the NHS. What are the key factors that create good communication?

6 Are you aware of the assumptions you make about people? To be consistently aware requires vigilance, reflective thinking and the ability to develop self-awareness. Think of the 'halo' effect and the 'horns' effect in psychology. The first suggests that if somebody makes a good impression, we are likely to attribute a range of good qualities, without any

demonstrable evidence of these. For example, at an interview, if you look smart, smile and speak well, you may be perceived as honest and trustworthy too. On the other hand, if you have a slouching manner and inappropriate eye contact, you might be seen as unacceptable. There is a sense in which patients and relatives are at an interview when they meet with healthcare professionals, particularly if they are on health service 'territory'. However sophisticated we are in our social behaviours, there is a residual 'animal' lying within, sensitive to the fact that we are not on home ground. It is worth remembering that however powerless we might feel at any point in our professional day, patients and relatives are more likely to feel at a disadvantage and to ascribe power, confidence and authority to us. We therefore have a responsibility, in the literal sense of that term, to respond to their needs.

7 Do you feel confident working in a multicultural society? Have you any other languages? Are there people you feel more or less comfortable with? Why?

8 Working on a children's ward means that you always have at least two patients – the child and the parent. They both need care, respect and clear communication. Reflect on your experience when there has been a conflict of interest between the child and the family. An example is Jehovah's Witnesses and their beliefs about blood transfusions.

9 The father wants to see a doctor for a diagnosis. This is perfectly understandable. Even at the end of the scenario, he only knows that Katya has had 'infections'. The hospital has a duty to inform clearly. As nurses may be doing diagnostic work in the future, how could the NHS convince the public that they will be as safe as doctors?

10 'Ethnic minority' is a divisive label and 'flying colours' has an upper middle class connotation. What do you think the ward staff will do when presented with the Polish food?

R is for Reason

'I'm running, running for my life. I abandon the car at the traffic lights in the middle of the city in the rush hour on a Friday night. I run into a shop. I know they'll think I'm mad if I say I'm looking for cover so I ask for the toilet instead. I run to the basement of the building. I get in the toilet. I lock the door. I collapse on the floor. What's happening to me?

I was on the way home from work and a lorry had swerved and nearly pushed me off a bridge over the motorway. I thought I was going to die. I was sure I was having a heart attack. I had been working on a building conservation project in Liverpool (I was an architect then) and these panic attacks had started whenever I had to climb a ladder to inspect the work. I just kept going to the GP for tranquillisers. She was happy to write 'stress' in my notes and to put me on repeat prescriptions.The tablets always warned me not to drive or operate machinery or have any alcohol but I had to keep driving for my job. And I often needed a stiff drink when I got in from work, just to unwind.

Then my mother died of a heart attack. I became convinced that my chest pains were serious. One night, I woke in such a state that I drove myself to the hospital. They put me on a heart monitor in A&E and reassured me that it was all in the mind. They had a trainee clinical psychologist on placement and he offered me some immediate help, sending me home with a 'thought diary' to complete. I had to record every trigger to the panic attacks over the next two weeks. How could I tell him that I didn't have time to be filling in a thought diary? I had a building project to complete. The symptoms got worse so I went back to the hospital and this time they sent me to a psychiatrist. He asked me questions about the relationship between my late mother and myself.

In less than an hour, he had implied that my mother had not really wanted me, and that her heart troubles had not been entirely physiological but more of a representation of an ambivalence towards both life and me. He suggested that I contact his secretary for a series of private appointments (at £65 an hour) to explore the problem in depth. He added, in a sonorous tone, that that would be the only way to get to the source of the pain and the resolution of my symptoms. I enquired about the availability of help on the NHS but the waiting list, he said, was six months long.

I was very unhappy. I went on the internet. There's psychiatry, psychology, psychotherapy, psychoanalysis and psychosynthesis. It was all very confusing. I was still convinced that I was not mad so I looked at alternatives. I found a long list of names of people who offered hypnotherapy, specifically for anxiety or phobias and panic attacks. I made several phone calls. The first sounded like she was overselling herself; I could barely get a word in edgeways. She insulted my intelligence by saying that she would not be turning me into a dancing chicken like a stage hypnotist. She also sounded hard and mean (she did not offer a brief initial consultation for free). The second one had a very relaxing voice and a very helpful manner, offering to send me a map of where she lived. We arranged a half-hour free appointment.

When I got there, there was a yapping terrier in the garden. The 'treatment' room was a spare bedroom and the woman herself seemed to be drunk. There were not any certificates on the walls; there were embroidered messages instead – *Life is beautiful ... I love my dog ... Why worry?*

Deciding to leave the free appointment increased my confidence, at least for a while. But the panic was still there and the insomnia was getting worse. I did not want to go back to the GP because I was trying to stop taking the drugs. Then an old friend visited and recommended a healer. At first I was not just sceptical but angry at the thought of meeting another unorthodox practitioner. But this person was different. She listened, I cried. She was gentle, I could trust her. She was generous with her time. We had tea together after two and a half hours. I had cried through a box of tissues. She had suffered too. She told me all about loss.'

Psychological issues

A panic attack is an experience of extreme terror; the fear is real but the reason is clouded and the awareness of the loss of reasoning increases the sense of fear. It may make people feel as if they are dying because of the increase in heart rate (due to anxiety) and the increased awareness of the heart's extra effort, which may convince people that they are about to have a heart attack. Unless experienced (or possibly, witnessed), it is difficult to understand how some situations can trigger such terror. Phobias (such as fear of heights which was a factor in this case) may create levels of anxiety approaching terror but a panic attack may feel like a 'close encounter' with death.

The conventional medical treatment for anxiety has not been helpful here. Repeat prescriptions are not doing anything to heal the pain. Further, the patient is contravening the safety requirements about not driving when drowsy.

The stress at work and driving to work, plus the development of vertigo leave him vulnerable to anxiety. Then he has a near-miss accident on the motorway and a full-blown panic attack. We might consider that the first panic attack can be the worst, in a way, than the second or third. Why? Because the person has not got a name for what is happening. They may have heard the term, but that is not the same as experiencing the sudden rush of terror. Once sensitised in this way, it can be very difficult to unpick the mental connections between the situation and the fear. It is like phobaphobia, or fear of fear.

The his mother dies. Fearful that he, too, is having a heart attack, he takes himself to A&E. It is interesting to note that he does not call the ambulance, so perhaps at one level he is able to reason that his problem is acute anxiety rather than imminent cardiac arrest. The 'thought diary' from the trainee clinical psychologist is not appropriate at this point. The psychiatrist makes things much worse and the effect of this lack of help pushes the patient towards whatever he can do for himself via the internet. Paradoxically, he gains strength from walking away from the dog-loving, drink-loving hypnotherapist. But without the good fortune of the visit from a friend, he would not have gone to the healer.

The giving of time, listening and tea contribute to the development of a dialogue between the two. They are equals in their common humanity and the patient feels healed (at least at that point in time). The healer tells him about her loss and it is as if they are enjoying the qualities of a good friendship. Crying is part of grieving; and for some people, the release of tears requires the consoling presence of another.

Personal and professional development

1 We are conditioned to living in a society where care has been 'professionalised'. Yet, in this example, some relief of pain is eventually achieved through the equivalent (though temporary) of friendship. What does this say about our social structures?

2 Repeat prescriptions of this kind are difficult to justify medically. Is there not a case, here, for primary care offering immediate access to some form of counselling? Or could health centres coordinate self-help groups for people suffering from work stress which is so common now?

3 Good interventions, particularly about emotional pain, have to be given at the right time and in the right way. The well-intended behaviourist suggestion about keeping a 'thought diary' did not help; the advice seemed like an extra burden. A&E staff can easily become limited to thinking in a crisis-interventionist way. What are the limitations of such an approach?

4 What gender did you attribute to the architect? Why?

5 Reflect on your experience of anxiety. Have you ever suffered a panic attack? Have you helped somebody with acute anxiety, phobias or panic?

6 Attitudes to psychiatry may be hard to shift; the fear of 'going mad' or being labelled 'mad' may linger in people's minds. There is considerable stigma towards mental illness, in spite of many attempts to inform the general public. Tabloid headlines about 'mad axe murderers' do not help; the popular Harry Potter books refer to some characters as 'mental' (*see* Introduction). This psychiatrist, sadly, would seem to have performed a mini-psychoanalysis on this patient, prior to suggesting *the only* way out of the pain is a series of expensive appointments. When people are vulnerable, the power of medical authority can be very strong. However, this patient turns away from the orthodox system and heads for hypnotherapy via the internet. How could the internet be rendered a safer resource?

7 The term 'healer' may have an old-fashioned ring to it. It also has a New Age connotation. What are your thoughts about 'healing gifts' and 'healing courses'?

8 'Prevention is better than cure.' How would you construct an in-house system to protect people from stress at work?

9 Ambivalent feelings in close relationships are not unusual. Reflect on your relationships with your mother, father, sisters, brothers, partner or friends. How would the loss of any of these people affect you?

10 We live in a time where accountability counts. The lack of an obvious path to complain about the inadequate hypnotherapist is not acceptable. Think about the heavily bureaucratised system of evaluation. How far do clinical protocols help or hinder the system of care?

S is for Status

'You know when you've made it. You've got a couple of BMWs (his and hers) tucked away in a triple garage, a runaround four-wheel on the driveway and a couple of bright kids at private schools. You've a Rolex on your wrist. You've got rid of the furniture. You've gone minimalist.

That's what I'd aimed for. That's what my wife and I had worked for. She'd been running a top-of-the-range nursery, taking children from three months old and I'd climbed the company ladder. We might not have managed the three cars or even the two kids (something wrong with Lauren's ovaries) but we were on our way in the dinner party circuit. We had budgeted to spend thousands on infertility treatment but the company renovating our second home in Tuscany had let us down badly.

I never thought that I'd have to go to the NHS for treatment. Until I was made redundant, we had private care. The consultant who did my first operation helped me in and out of my coat when I saw him in his study at home, the receptionist was charming, and before the operation itself, the anaesthetist came to my room to describe just what she would be doing. The room itself was beautifully decorated with all the facilities that you would expect from a good hotel.

Now, though, I am back in the hands of the state system. I can't believe the waiting times. I think I could stand that if the people were a bit more upbeat, not to mention bright. The last person who tended to me was a 'healthcare assistant' ... well ... I think that's what her badge said. You could hardly read it behind the mass of greasy hair. She was totally incoherent, said she'd go and ask somebody who 'knew what they were doing' and didn't return for at least half an hour. I wouldn't mind but I am a systems analyst and I think that they could have treated me as an intelligent person, not like the character in the next bed. I'd tried to start up a conversation with him but it was useless. I couldn't get a wink of sleep either. Just when you started to doze off in the early hours, the tea trolley rattled into sight. I tried to communicate with the nurses and other staff but they seemed to ignore me when I didn't laugh at their jokes. I'm not used to my bottom being called a 'bum' and being told I'll have a 'numb bum' after the pre-med. I didn't want one anyway as I prefer to remain alert as I'm wheeled to theatre. I want to know exactly what's going on and I want to have my say.

I'm not prepared to say what, precisely, is wrong with me. I have always enjoyed good health until recently. I eat all the right things, I do not drink and I play competitive sports at least three times a week. I do not have time for a social life as such. I was brought up to be a high flyer and I was flying high until the company was taken over. It wasn't the loss of the job so much as the perks. I had my own parking space with my name on it and I had been led to believe that a directorial position was imminent. I've always been single-minded and goal-orientated. How will I cope with the loss of status at the golf club?

As an afterthought, I should add that there was little difference in the quality of *medical* care between the private and public sectors. My over-worked GP had made sure that I had had all the necessary tests which probably saved my life.'

Psychological issues

This patient's expectations have been disappointed. He is experiencing unexpected loss of health and the loss of status formerly attributed to him through both his work role and the private health system. He does, however, begrudgingly admit that the medical care has been acceptable under the NHS.

His experience of the healthcare assistant's self-presentation and inadequate communication skills contributes to his dissatisfaction. He is also subjected to a public ward, lack of sleep and medical humour, which he finds unacceptable.

He is unwilling to tell us from what disease he is suffering. It is as if he feels personally responsible for the failure of his body to act like a functioning part, a necessary element in his ambitious lifestyle.

He minds that he is no longer part of private healthcare. Even before he meets the healthcare assistant (with the perceived poor hygiene in the form of greasy hair), he is biased in his thinking, ostensibly due to the waiting times but we can infer that it is the loss of status as well.

Is it morally justifiable to have any system of healthcare that divides the rich from the poor?

We live in an image-conscious society, dominated by glossy marketing materials which try and lure us to believe that the image is the reality. Critic-ally evaluate some of the advertisements for private healthcare. Are they offering more style than substance?

This patient is deliberately designed to be hard to like. Loss of status, compared with loss of life, limb, sight, friend, pet, home, money, car keys, etc., could be difficult to sympathise with, and yet in our society, for some people, their status is their identity and their identity depends on their status.

Personal and professional development

1 Reflect on your attitude to status. What sort of status symbols do you own? Does it matter, for example, whether your car has an up-to-date number plate? Do you like wearing clothes that show the designer's name, even if this means that you are effectively advertising for the company?

2 Is it a basic human right to access free healthcare at the point of delivery?

3 Attribution theory suggests that we attribute qualities (good and bad) according to the impression people make.[1] If we see somebody behaving badly (as in this scenario) we are more likely to attribute character deficits to the person than to allow for the fact that the situation could be the main cause. This is known as the primary attribution error. Considering hospitals are likely to make people uneasy, reflect on your approach to people who are unpleasant if not rude to deal with. Are you inclined to attribute some sort of blame first or are you able to think of a range of factors that may contribute to irritability?

4 The healthcare assistant conveys poor personal hygiene and her badge is unreadable. She is a poor communicator and, crucially, does not return with information within an appropriate amount of time. Reflect on your communication skills and self-presentation.

5 Do you think that people who look after themselves well (as in this case) should be afforded a system of 'credits', which might be used to move them more quickly up a waiting list?

6 Equally, do you think that services should be rationalised against helping heavy smokers who do not exercise and eat meaty diets?

7 Status reflects social position and this man is fearful of his place at the golf club, having been made redundant. The health service is hierarchical in its structure, more status being ascribed to consultants than cleaners, and yet, as in this example, the perception of good hygiene is a step towards trust. If you were to rearrange the health service, how would you re-distribute status?

8 Do you have any private healthcare?

9 To what extent do you think dentists are justified in leaving the NHS?

10 Have you worked in both private and public sectors? What are your observations about the similarities and differences in the medical care?

Reference

1 Rungapadiachy D (1999) *Interpersonal Communication and Psychology for Health Care Professionals.* Butterworth-Heinemann, Oxford.

T is for Trust

'When I first found the lump, I panicked. It was just on the edge of my vagina. And I didn't want to go to the GP because he was a man and I didn't feel confident enough to ask to see a woman. I was only 19 years old, new to the area and I was scared that they'd ask me questions about 'safe sex'. I'd been abused by my dad growing up; not as bad as sexual intercourse but from about the age of six he'd make me lie down with him after school 'for a bit of a cuddle'. Sometimes he'd touch me where I knew he shouldn't but when I told my mum she got very cross and said that children who lie go blind.

I didn't have any friends to talk to. I went back to the receptionist at the health centre to get an appointment but she looked very busy. She didn't smile and when I finally got her attention, I nearly dried up. "You want to see a *lady* doctor, is that it?" But when I went through, the doctor was very nice. She said it was a Bartholin cyst (not cancer as I'd feared) and that it would clear up with antibiotics. She seemed to sense that there was something else on my mind and offered me an appointment the following week. I went back and she took the time to listen. When she said I could do with counselling, I wanted to ask her if I could just keep seeing her every week. Fortunately the counsellor was too booked-up to fit me in and so the doctor said she'd see me every week at the end of surgery.

It made such a difference just knowing that weekly appointment was there, like an anchor.

I got myself on a part-time computing course at the local college and found a flat to share. My appointments with the doctor got shorter and shorter; it was just really a few minutes' encouragement. She really increased my confidence when she said that I looked a bit like her daughter who was going off to university.

Months went by. The receptionist sometimes gave me these funny looks, looks which said: You shouldn't be taking up so much time.

Then I missed two periods. I went to see the doctor rather than paying for the test at Boots The Chemist. The receptionist glared at me through the gap in the window. "Your doctor", she said, "Your doctor is on sick leave herself".

I asked when she would be back and I was told that she would only be part-time in the future but that I could see the locum if I needed to. I know it's silly but I felt let down and betrayed. When I got home, my flatmate was out.

There was a text message on my mobile phone from Ben, ending the relationship. I didn't know what to do. I rang one of those numbers to see if I could get a termination but there was just an answerphone. I wasn't going to become a single parent. I ran to Boots, just before it was closing at six, and spent my last bit of money on a pregnancy test. The pharmacist was old enough to be my mother and although she looked concerned, I wasn't going to admit to her the difficulty I was in.

The test was positive. I went to the pub. My flatmate wasn't there. I took my card and drew out the last bit of money and spent it on vodka and crisps. I drank myself to sleep. I woke up sick. I went out to the shops and ran into the pharmacist who was so kind that I burst into tears. She bought me a coffee and I started to tell her everything. She said that she would help me make the right decision.'

Psychological issues

Trust is the basis of any relationship. Sexual abuse, perhaps from the sensationalised reports in some parts of the press or media, may be immediately conceived in our minds as intercourse between fathers, stepfathers, etc. and daughters. But inappropriate touch is a betrayal of trust. Not being believed (by her mother) is an added blow to any sense of self-worth. How do we build up trust? Over time. It is not an instant gift of gold; the precious metal needs proving within the furnace of change, as the knowledge of one person by another grows. Trust is always risky. Obviously people in authority, such as parents and healthcare professionals, have to be particularly careful.

This patient is inherently vulnerable because of her background, age and present circumstances. We could also argue that she is more vulnerable to the breakdown of trust in a society that moves at such a pace that relationships may not have time to form. 'Moving on' is a phrase commonly heard and accepted, not just about geographical shifts but about leaving some 'friends' or contacts behind. Questions like 'Are you *in* a relationship at the moment?' add to the feeling of friendship being a temporary thing. The word 'in' implies its opposite, 'out', subtly suggesting that if you are not 'in' one, you are in some way excluded. This may be a reason why there is so much social pressure on people to stay in unhealthy relationships.

The doctor, it could be argued, goes beyond the call of duty by offering the structure of regular weekly appointments. The receptionist implies to the patient that she is partly to blame for the doctor's stress and that from now on, only a locum will be available. The pharmacist gives time and consideration to the girl's problems. The pregnancy advisory service only has an answerphone. What should have happened in this situation?

Do you think we could do more to protect teenagers from unwanted pregnancies? Where does the responsibility lie?

Standing at reception in a health centre or speaking in a pharmacy can be difficult as privacy may be compromised. Teenagers are likely to experience times of painful self-consciousness. Is this an argument for running services specifically for certain age groups?

Medical receptionists are often vilified in films and entertainment. The unsmiling head at the window, wearing unattractive spectacles and presenting obstacles to access to healthcare is a stereotypical image. Are they hindered by relatively low pay, relatively low status or the common occupational stress of running two information systems (paper and computer) at once? How could their morale be lifted?

We are living in the 'age of anxiety'. Trust at the micro (broken relationships) and the macro (cynicism about politics and the representation of these in the media) levels is under threat.[1] For an excellent review of the wider issues facing a society in a spin about 'spin', the Reith lectures (2002) on trust can be read on the BBC Radio Four website.[2]

Personal and professional development

1 Reflect on trust. Think of times when you have gained and lost trust, both in a personal and professional context. If multidisciplinary teams have broken down, how have you rebuilt trust?

2 Therapeutic touch can play a large part in developing a sense of care and trust. Design a short programme teaching the appropriate use of touch between patients and professionals where they are of opposite gender.

3 If you are a practice manager (or any manager of staff), how would you develop (and sustain) the social skills of receptionists to be both welcoming and, when necessary, assertive?

4 We live in a sexualised society (*see* page 17). This means that social pressure steadily exerts itself on everyone to think that everyone else is enjoying an active if not adventurous sex life. What sort of realistic health campaign could be run to protect teenagers? Design a poster, for example one with a young teenager unhappily pregnant and sucking her thumb.

5 Imagine you were the pharmacist in this scenario. What sort of advice would you give this girl? The girl describes the pharmacist as saying that she will help her decide what to do. Is this really what happened do you think?

6 In what ways do you agree or disagree with the doctor giving extra time to this patient?

7 Reflect on the ethical issues surrounding pregnancy and abortion.

8 Imagine you are a nurse working for NHS Direct and you receive a phone call from a young girl fearful that she is pregnant. She tells you that her partner has just ended the relationship and that she only has a bottle of vodka for comfort. The line suddenly goes dead. The next caller is an abusive male. Your shift ends and you go home only to discover that your partner has been having an affair. How would you begin to sift through these feelings?

9 Beginning relationships of trust are part of what good healthcare is all about. Do you think enough care and attention is paid to the ending or closure of these?

10 Where do you see yourself in terms of trust:

- Trusting?
- Trustworthy?
- Dependable?
- Reliable?
- Naïve?
- Cynical?
- Bitter?
- Cautious?
- Open?
- Closed?

References

1 Smith R (2004) Transparency: a modern essential. *BMJ*: **328**(7448): 0–f.

2 www.bbc.co.uk/radio4/reith2002

U is for Understanding

'We lost our daughter. Hospital error. Enquiry. What's the point?

She'd just come back from celebrating her 18th birthday on holiday in Ibiza and all that was wrong with her was an insect bite. But it turned septic and she had to be taken in. We'll never know what went wrong but somehow the information got lost in the system, the information that she was allergic to penicillin.* She suffered a heart attack and ended up in a coma for two years. Finally, my wife and I had to make the decision to switch off the life support system.

Our adopted son, Mark is training to be a legal executive, specialising in accidental injury. He wants us to sue the hospital trust. My wife has been unable to make any decisions since the day our daughter died. I have to do everything. We are now a family torn apart. I've always seen myself as a laid-back realist. What happened, happened. Legal wrangling won't bring her back. Mark and Sarah never got on but he's adopting some sort of crusader-spirit now and says he's going to get that hospital.

The enquiry produced an apology and the spokesman for the Trust offered the most sincere condolences and reassured us that lessons had been learnt. That day I was in my office (I'm in building supplies) and the quote on the calendar read: "Something explained, something endured, something forgiven, something cured". I nearly broke down.

It's five years on now. My wife remains stuck in the past. She's sometimes so indecisive she is rooted to the floor in the kitchen unable to decide whether she's going to the fridge or the cooker. I persuaded her to get help but nothing seems to change. Mark agreed with me in the end that there was no point in pursuing the hospital. But he doesn't bother to come home any more.

---

* (A year later) 'We think we've just found out what really happened. It looks like a foreign nurse had done the admissions paperwork and taken Sarah's case history. Sarah had told her, we think, about her allergy to penicillin. Maybe the nurse didn't have good enough English. Then there was a shift change and somebody else was supposed to put the information on to a database.

We got the update from a researcher who is doing a longitudinal study on hospital accountability. He told us that things had got worse in the last 10 years. He said that there was a lot less rigour now in the way information is collected on admission.'

We had a terrible row. We said terrible things. He threatened to go and find his real mother.

I'm not so well myself. I just don't understand how this could have happened to us. We were happy. I want to throw the family photos away, those reminders of better days. But every time I go to the bin, my wife stays me with that look of hers, which seems to be blaming me not just for being a workaholic but for being alive.'

Psychological issues

The loss of a child, at any age, cuts through our expectations. We expect our children to outlive us. The loss of understanding, the disbelief that such a series of errors could lead to the death of a young girl just about to embark on adult life is understandable. It is clear from the tone of this scenario that apologies from the hospital trust mean very little when trust has been betrayed. It is also clear that the older adults, the 'biological' parents of the girl realise that no amount of legal action or compensation would ever be worth all the effort. Money does not replace people.

The family is torn apart. We have the parents rendered incommunicative. We have the shift from sibling rivalry to sudden crusading and there is the interesting fact that the brother is adopted. He is threatening to seek his birth mother, and in so doing, possibly raising more feelings of loss in the parents.

There is the decision to switch off the life support system. Is it surprising that the mother is traumatised into deep indecisiveness, even over small decisions in the kitchen, years later? The husband perceives that the wife blames him, as he, in his grief, tries to throw the past away by throwing away the family photographs. Why should we assume that people grieve in the same way? Grief forces the person to turn away, in some way, and at some point, from the moment of loss. We talk about 'letting go' but the timing and the way in which this is done is an individual thing.

At the beginning of the 21st century, we talk a lot about stress. It is common to say amongst friends, family and colleagues that we are feeling stressed. Are we less likely to admit to *feeling lost*, or to grieve openly about our losses (*see* the Introduction — 'the stiff upper lip')? We are also living with two information systems (paper and technology) running alongside. In this tragic case, it is possible that confusions occurred in both.

Years on, the family is still interested in trying to find out what happened. The researcher digs up the fact that a foreign nurse may have been the starting point of the confusion by her lack of understanding of the word 'penicillin'. How can patients be safeguarded against healthcare professionals whose first language is not English?

We all want to understand or make sense of life; our brains are designed to recognise patterns and forms. We do not like chaos and the feelings of loss of control that go with it. However, we are living at a time when more changes have taken place in the social structures of our globe in the last 50 or so years, than in the hundreds of years before. What effect does this have on our consciousness?

Personal and professional development

1 Reflect on your experience of errors in healthcare. Have you ever been in the awkward position of 'whistleblower' or stuck in the dilemma of what to say or whether to say anything?
2 Put yourself in the shoes of the foreign nurse. Imagine trying to take a case history on a busy ward with uncertain English. Design a training programme for the updating of language skills for E2L clinicians.
3 'Something explained, something endured, something forgiven, something cured.' Sometimes the best psychology is found in the simplest forms. How would you help a man to feel comfortable about crying?
4 Supposing you had to counsel parents facing the decision to switch off the life support system. How would you start this process and how would you end it?
5 What experience do you have working with adopted children and stepchildren? How different do you think the bonds of family attachment are, depending on the biological origin of children?
6 Reflect on your family of origin. Do the verses below apply?

The Sibriv	**Family: anagrammatic effects**
Here is a song that I give	I am 'Fly'
To you about the dreaded Sibriv	Am I 'Fly'?
It affects us all, well nearly most	"Fly!" I am ...
The brother or sister who	May I fly?
horribly boasts	
But don't be sad or mad or green	Fly aim?
With envy for the depressing fiend	I ...
It's only full of froth and spittle	
Very small very little.	

7 The law and medicine have become more entwined recently. What are the advantages and disadvantages of this?

8 The word 'decision' comes from the Latin, *cedere*, to slay. Think of the last decision you made. To what extent did you feel that you had to slay the alternative course of action?

9 The family is one of our oldest institutions and yet it is under threat. How could the government help support family life?

10 What are your views on euthanasia?

V is for Voice

'I'm a nursing student and I've chosen to specialise in 'learning disabilities'. It's probably because my best friend at school was 'special needs' and when I was in Year 12, I chose to help at a young disabled unit, helping them to ride horses.

It's strange on my course. There are four 'branches' in nursing:

- adult
- child
- mental health
- learning disabilities.

It's as if the students and their tutors almost represent the branches themselves. For example, the adult branch being the largest group, adopt the ways of any majority group in society. The child branch tutors seem to be a bit childish themselves. One of the students said a tutor had made them sit in silence for being late, and on another occasion, a tutor had made a student stand outside because her mobile phone had gone off. Then the minority groups (mental health and learning disabilities) seem to have less status, but in very subtle ways. It makes me cross that a university should reinforce the sort of stigma that goes on in society anyway. Universities are about teaching people to think, I think. What other institution in society has this responsibility?

Nursing is really a practical, hands-on job. I'm not sure that it should be a degree course in a university. Nursing is about caring and you can care whether or not you can write and reference an essay. I do think it is important that people are taught to think clearly and rigorously but it seems to be much more of a political move than an educational one, putting nursing students in universities. They think that we have to be the same as doctors, somehow. Is that just to get us better pay or better status, or both? Or is it to devolve some of the responsibilities of doctors to us? Also, I've realised why the school of healthcare studies is in such a mess. It's because it has three masters:

- the university (which emphasises the academic side)
- the NHS trusts (which want nurses who can *do* the job)

- the Nursing and Midwifery Council (which wants to keep control of the curriculum, amongst other things).

Where are the needs of patients in all this? Why do they have to keep changing the way nurses are trained? When my mum was training, they were really careful about hygiene but now people have a greater risk of catching infections when they are *in* hospital!

It is frustrating on placements to have to wear the badge, *student* nurse, because that makes me feel that I don't really have a voice. And if any group needs a nurse-with-a-voice, it must be those people who have no voice at all – people with learning disabilities. I know it's necessary to distinguish me from the qualified staff for the sake of visitors, but I am a mature student with a lot of experience who feels held back by some of the petty procedures (and thinking).

This perception was brought home to me on my last placement. One of the 'clients' (and that sounds like a customer in a hairdressing salon), a Down's syndrome man, had been given the news that his aunt had died. Everyone was fussing around him and there was a lot of concern that he understood what death really meant. That is something else that I have noticed, fussing is not the same as caring. Also, assumptions are made all the time about what our 'clients' do and do not understand. I am convinced that nobody can say for sure what is going on in *any* person's mind, whether or not they are disabled. As the day of the funeral approached, the Home made plans for him to attend. He had worked on a picture of his aunt which he wanted to have placed on the coffin before the service. I was so upset the next time I saw him, upset because he was so upset. The Home had changed the plan at the last minute, as they could not get sufficient cover for him to attend. He had put on his suit and he was refusing to remove his suit and everyone was getting uptight because they could not make him get changed. I could stand back from the situation and see what was going on, but I did not really have the professional status to be heard, and when you are a student you always have this slight fear at the back of your mind that if you rock the boat you may not get a good report. I would have been happy to have come in and taken the man to his aunt's funeral. If I'd been on an 'apprenticeship' type of training, that could well have happened.'

Psychological issues

The loss of voice in this scenario is the loss within the clinical context; the nurse clearly has ideas of her own which she can express fluently and assertively. The patient with Down's syndrome may not have as clear a voice but he is demonstrating by his refusal to get changed that he is frustrated and upset that he cannot attend his aunt's funeral. So there are two losses of voice here and there is also the *lack* of opportunity in the Home: the lack of encouragement to speak up and to be heard.

The issue of how to train nurses is raised:

- points about the differences between training (for a practical skill) and education (for thinking)
- the confusion between academic and clinical skills
- the similarities and differences between doctors and nurses in a system which is increasingly passing some of the former responsibilities from doctors to nurses.

Dissatisfaction with pettiness both within the course and the clinical context is expressed. Recognition that good thinking skills are necessary, but that they do not necessarily have to be assessed by essay-writing assignments. Finally, the comment is made that an apprenticeship-type programme could have been the answer to the meeting of the patient's needs in this case.

The wearing of a student nurse badge when a mature student is described as a contributory factor to the loss of voice. Further the fear of being marked down limits this student's intelligent approach. Institutionalisation is an insidious process. How can its power be limited, whilst safeguarding the structures it protects?

The perception that caring does not have to be fussy is a good one. The moment when the staff are getting uptight because the patient will not get changed is an example. Confrontations and coercions are rarely the best approach to take because they set up an 'us' and 'them' situation. We get the impression that the patient is winning some kind of power game, and we can reflect on the paradox that the disabled person is 'winding up' the 'abled' staff. Resolution of conflict needs to be 'win–win' for the preservation of everyone's dignity.

Personal and professional development

1 Reflect on times when you feel that you have not been able to speak up, either as a student or a professional, or in your personal life. What does it feel like – *loss of voice*? Or would you say that you suffer from a *lack of voice*? In other words, you think that you have never really had the chance to speak up for yourself, or you think that you have nothing to

say, or perhaps you are scared that you do not know how to express certain things.

2 Think about the training of healthcare professionals.[1] How would you improve the education and training of doctors, nurses, dentists, pharmacists, chiropodists, homeopaths, etc.? What is the difference between 'education' and 'training'?

3 How would you have dealt with this situation differently? Think of the man with Down's syndrome sitting in his suit, refusing to get changed.

4 What do you think about badges? Are labels of this kind necessary or useful? If nurses wear the word 'student' when training, should registrars be identified as trainee consultants?

5 What do you think are the advantages and disadvantages of dividing nursing training into four branches? Do you think that evidence-based assessment of really good nurses, followed by apprenticeship of students to them would be a good idea?

6 How would you explain death to somebody with limitations on their intelligence?

7 Do you agree that it is impossible to assume what is going on inside anybody's mind? If so, can you proceed via tentative hypotheses? That is, you are aware of your hunches and assumptions and test each one out, first of all in your own mind.

8 Think of status differentials in the health service, an obvious one being the gap between consultant and hospital porter, for example. What are the advantages and disadvantages of hierarchical systems?

9 Think about empowerment. Power is concomitant with responsibility. How often do you see too much power with too little responsibility being exercised? Equally, are there occasions where staff have too much responsibility and insufficient power?

10 Think about 'patients as partners' as rhetoric and as reality.

References

1 Newton L (1981) In defense of the traditional nurse. *Nursing Outlook*. **29**(6): 348–54.

W is for Wife

'People assume I left my wife but that's not true. She made me go. She was having a breakdown of some sort, a mid-life crisis, they said. Our son was only three. He told me why she'd made me go: "Because you didn't mow the lawn." And now I'm the one under a psychiatrist while my wife has kept the marital home, bought me out and tried to turn the children against me.

I came into hospital voluntarily. I just didn't think I could go on. I'd been staying in bed all day for nearly a year, living off burgers in a bedsit and the school where I taught had told me that they had to let me go. I didn't expect the place to be this bad; I'd read articles in the *Guardian* about the lack of asylum in asylums but this place is unbelievable. There is nothing for us to do. The patients are just left pretty much to themselves, especially at weekends when the loss strikes the hardest. I've lost the sense of future that people who are married take for granted. I've lost all sense of structure. The weekends used to be easy. We had a pattern we lived by. I've lost all sense of belonging. I'd only ever wanted to be a family man but my wife said that she was sick of 'domestickity'. "All I ever do is mow the lawns! All I ever do is clean up after all of you!", she'd cried, before pouring red wine over my head and ripping off the parish priest's cross when he came to visit us to try and mediate.

Most of the other patients are chain smokers. There's this really nice woman, Ruth, who cracked up working as a drug rep. She couldn't cope with being a 'drug pusher' anymore she said, especially after the only thing that had ever helped her with depression was a homeopathic remedy. At first I thought she was mad (not just sad, like most of us in here) when she said the remedy had given her an insight: *There's a whole world outside your head.* I was a science teacher and the idea that a small white sugary pill could give healing insights was a bit much. But, as she put it, the insight started her on a long journey out of 'the black hole'. She really tries to see the world as it is: the world outside her own thoughts. But this psychiatric ward is so depressing. You feel like a weary blood clot travelling through the veins of a geriatric body, when you walk around the corridors. And, of course, you never get any sleep. Everybody is so drugged up, they are straining to breathe at night and the snoring makes sleep impossible.

Ruth and I talk to each other a lot. We were comparing notes about the staff the other day. She'd been told that she had manic depression by her psychiatrist. He's a national expert on the disease, but when she asked him to tell her what he knew, he retorted "You wouldn't understand!" She'd done a psychology degree in her twenties. Putting herself in hospital was a hard decision, because whilst she knew the research on their inadequacy, she also knew that she needed time away from home. Her CPN (community psychiatric nurse), an attractive young man, had told her that he found vulnerable women attractive. We did not know whether he was trying to be kind, to boost her morale, but it did not seem appropriate. The staff have also assumed that because Ruth and I spend time together, we must be falling in love and they keep teasing us about wedding bells. It's just the loss of identity as half-of-a-couple that's been getting to me.

None of our friends or relatives come to visit us. They're ashamed, embarrassed or scared of this place. Or perhaps they just feel helpless in the face of depression. We all stick together as a group of patients. We have our own little community really – the sleepers, the smokers, the ranters, the ravers. You try and help others along the way, making a coffee in the knifeless stainless steel kitchen, persuading the odd obsessive-compulsive that there are no drawing pins in the sugar bowl, nor monsters in the swing bin.

A while ago an anorexic girl was sectioned. She'd told the OT (occupational therapist) that she didn't think she could go on, and the OT, without her permission, had told one of the nurses. He read the legal stuff gleefully and she broke down in floods of tears. Fearful that this stain would be on her record forever, desperate that this would stop her getting a job, she ran to her bed and got hold of her nail file, which she had hidden under the mattress. When Ruth and I found her, she was cutting herself again.'

Psychological issues

The key issue here is the state of 'mental' health services. We have three characters:

- a divorced man
- a depressed drug representative
- an anorexic.

None of their needs are being met by the system. They are forming an informal group of community support. It is interesting that the man's wife is perceived to be having a breakdown and yet she is not receiving help.

There are four examples of bad professional practice:

- the arrogance of the consultant (based on false assumptions about the educational status of his patient)
- the lack of confidentiality between the OT and the ward nurse
- the reference to attraction to vulnerable patients by the CPN
- the seeming delight in the exercise of power by the nurse who 'sections' the anorexic girl.

There are basic gaps in the physical care – smokers and snorers. There is the specific reference to the poor quality of facilities at the weekends, just when the man feels he is at his most vulnerable. He is struggling with a multiplicity of losses and the assumption by the staff that he is trying to replace the main loss by 'falling in love' with Ruth is unfounded. Joking about 'wedding bells', whilst well meant perhaps, is insensitive.

Homeopathy has helped Ruth. We have an ex-science teacher and a drug representative possibly having some of their fundamental beliefs challenged.

The physical restrictions of the buildings are described – dark corridors and airlessness.

The innocence of the man's three-year-old son provides a contrast to the realities of the situation in which these adults find themselves.

The priest, in his attempt at reconciliation, finds himself stripped of his cross.

Personal and professional development

1 What is your experience of psychiatric care, in hospitals and the community? How typical is this account? Have you read the Patients' Charter outlining the expectations of care?
2 Make a list of all the factors contributing to the depression in the two main characters. Where would you start to change the hospital's contribution?
3 Critically evaluate the Mental Health Act, sectioning and the power it gives to the staff.
4 What do you make of homeopathy and other complementary medicines in the treatment of emotional problems?
5 Design a therapeutic weekend for these patients within the constraints of the hospital.
6 Revise your reading and thinking about depression – its causes and treatments.

7 Divorce (and this man is a Catholic) is riddled with loss:

- of the sense of future
- of what might have been
- of identity as half-of-a-couple
- of self-confidence.

How could the NHS structure services appropriate to the needs of men and women going through this process? Divorce has, after all, reached 'epidemic' proportions according to many articles in the daily press.

8 The patients have formed their own community. To what extent do you think this sense of community is healing in itself, and what are its drawbacks?

9 Gender is a factor in this scenario. We have the comments from the CPN and we have the staff's assumptions about the man and Ruth 'falling in love' just because they are spending time together. What does this say about (a) our sexualised society and (b) unthinking comments made by staff? Would it be better if gender were only on the agenda in bed, just before bed and just after bed within the privacy of people's homes?

10 Have you ever been depressed or tried to help somebody with depression?[1] What sort of feelings did you experience and what helped you the most? You might like to look at the literature that stresses that a mismatch between the inner values a person holds and the work they do may be a major cause of stress. Ruth has been helped by homeopathy and yet she is being forced to sell drugs as a 'rep', which is a job involving considerable stress such as driving on motorways, facing receptionists who may or may not be feeling receptive and having to reach targets. Interestingly, as this book goes to press, the government is trying to persuade doctors to prescribe less drugs in an attempt to keep costs (to the NHS) down! There are also worrying changes in the law about power and control over patients in psychiatric facilities.

Useful tip
Contact MIND (www.mind.org.uk) if you are concerned about poor care in a psychiatric facility.

Reference

1 Stewart G (2000) *Understanding Mental Illness.* MIND publications, London.

X is for Xmas

'I'm 85 years old this December and still in the flats. I've a good life. I like to have a bath on a Saturday night with a nice drink, a packet of chocolates and a good book. I just soak for a couple of hours. The district nurse said I should have one of those disabled showers now because I could get stuck in the bath. But I don't like to be a bother.

I'm what they call a 'walking miracle'. My heart's gone, my blood's thin and I've got a big growth on my liver. They said they could go in but it wasn't worth it. And anyway I couldn't leave my budgies with nobody to look after them. I can still just about walk to the shops and the café for a brew. I haven't a lot of hurry left in me.

It's just Christmas that can get you down. I never trouble the neighbours usually, but I give them a card on the Eve, late on, so they don't think I'm after one back. They're not very friendly at the best of times. I have told them how to bring their kiddies up, just little things like saying 'hello' and 'good-bye' instead of the grunts I usually get. But they swore at me and then one of their lads tried to run me over with his skateboard.

Christmas morning, I like to get up early and treat myself to a turkey bap. Then I walk to the telephone and if it hasn't been vandalised I try and phone my gentleman friend that I met at the café. It's not easy because he is married and his wife can get very jealous, but then I've always had a very nice pair of legs.

Christmas dinner, I have a boil-in-a-bag beef and Yorkshire pudding, then a small brandy and a packet of cigarettes. You still can't beat the first draw on a fag. I don't care what they say, my grandad swore by smoking and he lived to 90 years old.

Christmas afternoon, I turn up the gas fire for a bit of a treat, let the birds out of their cage and watch the Queen with Rex balanced on my finger.

Then it's nearly done with. Boxing Day is best spent in bed and then it's not that long until the New Year. This year, Frank promised me that he would call round at midnight. He said he'd pretend he had to take the dog out but he didn't arrive until one in the morning. He suddenly felt really poorly. I said I'd ring for the doctor but he said we couldn't put them out on New Year. But when I tried to get through I got connected to one of these call centres. She was called Charlene and she didn't sound very caring for an out-of-hours doctors' service. Just when I thought I'd sorted out an appointment, she told me it had gone off her computer screen. Frank was outside the phone box saying his chest pains were getting worse and he was turning a funny colour. I was getting flustered and cross so I started telling Charlene what I thought of her. She told us to ring 999 and get an ambulance if it was really an emergency. So I did. Before they even got to us, I'd stuffed a couple of aspirin down him as you're supposed to do. I couldn't face ringing his wife. The paramedics were very understanding. They injected him with this 'thrombolitic' thingy and drove him away in the ambulance. I was left with the dog and trying to think of what to say to Elsie, his wife.'

Psychological issues

In this scenario, there is a tension between the cheerfulness of the 85-year-old woman and her circumstances. There is also romance over a certain age. The paramedics are described as being understanding and yet we do not know what it is they understand – Frank's heart trouble, Frank's visit to a woman who is not his wife on New Year's Day, the difficulty the 85-year-old woman has had in trying to access the right sort of healthcare?

There is the poor diet, beliefs about smoking being safe, the lack of appropriate washing facilities and the sense of resigned loneliness at Christmas. The lack of community spirit in the flats is made clear by the episodes with neighbours, as well as the possibility of the public telephone having been vandalised.

Charlene, the operative at the call centre is perceived to be unhelpful. She may have been attempting to be informative about the loss of the appointment on her computer screen, but from the perspective of old age in a telephone box (with a friend outside the box showing signs of increasing difficulty), it is not surprising that the old lady became frustrated and angry. Frank had not wanted to disturb the doctor at New Year and yet he ends up in an ambulance after a 999 call. His lady friend is left with the problem of his dog and the fact that his wife, Elsie, does not know of her existence. It might be interesting to speculate on how these problems are solved.

Pets are providing important relationships in this scenario. The lady cannot go into hospital because she does not want to leave her budgies and the man has been able to use his dog as an excuse to go out for a walk and see his friend on New Year's Eve.

Personal and professional development

1 Reflect on your experience of caring for the elderly. How typical is this unwillingness to disturb the doctor?

2 Think about Christmas and the range of emotional reactions at this time of year. Design a **Prevention of Loneliness** health campaign for the week from Christmas to the New Year.

3 Does it strike you as strange, the possibility of romantic or sexual relationships between men and women in their 80s? How can ageist attitudes be prevented in the health system?

4 It could be argued that the elderly need high frequency but low intensity and low duration contacts to prevent loneliness; how can these needs be met by nursing (and other) staff? Or is it really a question of re-creating community spirit in our towns and cities?

5 Research the effect of out-of-hours doctors' services on physical and psychological health. How can call centres and computer screens be humanised?

6 Think about your own use of the telephone in delivering any sort of advice about health. How could it be improved?

7 Would you try and persuade this woman to change her diet and to give up smoking?

8 Reflect on your experience of Christmas. Do you spend it with people who you choose or do you feel that you are under pressure to spend three days with relatives in a fug of central heating, television, turkey and drink?

9 Medicine prides itself on *doing* something to help people get better from illness. There is very little to do for this woman as she has decided not to have an operation for the growth on her liver because she cannot leave her budgies. How do you feel when faced with problems that do not have obvious clinical solutions? How comfortable are you just *being* with a patient?

10 Relationships matter. Rex, the budgerigar may not be the greatest company. On the other hand, he could be comforting to talk to and might have the advantage of not having a lot to say back. What effect has the loss of pets in your life had on your well-being?

Y is for the Y-chromosome

'I'm an engineer but I've lost my momentum. I used to be happy working at the brewery in Tadcaster, but since my partner dumped me everything's gone wrong. I was made redundant and then my blood pressure shot up with the pressure of trying to get another job at 40 plus. The doctor put me on ACE inhibitors in a three-minute consultation. I couldn't tell her about my willy wilting all over the place, could I? One of the blokes at the brewery had tried to see his doctor with willy trouble last year and he told us that she'd said she'd have to get her microscope out to find it. What's wrong with women? Haven't they got any sensitivity? Don't they realise that a man *is* his sexual performance?

I went on the internet. The porn sites. I pictured the next lot of interviewers in leatherette bondage being chastised by brewery workers, but it didn't help. I neither got the job nor any activation on the willy front. Talking of fronts, I discarded the Y-fronts and invested in a bargain bag of boxers made out of some sort of slippery silk, but they got mangled up in the launderette and I was too embarrassed to claim them. Then, I ordered a vacuum pump off the internet, but when it arrived I'm sure the postman knew what it was because it wouldn't fit through the letterbox so I had to go and claim it from the post office. When I unpacked it and tried to read the instructions I was nearly sick. The next thing I did was buy '*Loaded*'. It was threatening at first because all the models had six-pack musculature, but I read the columns carefully. It made me realise just how naff my technique had been. It told me how to wiggle and twirl my tongue around the ladies' navels and how to listen to what they had to say. It did warn me that women use sentences in bed instead of the little mewing noises that we guys like, and that in itself cheered me up. It brought back that little spark of aggression that can really help a bloke get and sustain an erection.

But once I was back out in the field, on the pull, it all came to nothing, so it was back to the internet. This time I tried the NHS site. It told me that my medication could be the reason why I was having trouble. Women doctors! Then it said you could have sexual counselling. I've never seen myself as a muesli-man and the thought of going to some head-nodding, middle-aged woman with grey hair did not appeal. I rang the surgery to see if I could have an appointment with the practice nurse. I thought that just being with her in her little office might be the stimulus to get me going. But when I arrived and saw her, I pretended I just wanted my blood pressure checked. She said it was nearly normal and that the ACE inhibitors were doing the trick. She paused and with a knowing look, asked me if everything was all right in the 'other department'. There was no way I could admit it to this blonde bombshell.

The next time I was visiting my sister, I tried a bit of banter with her husband – joking about willies and middle age and liking a drink and trying to suss what his 'other department' was up to. But he didn't get what I was on about. I went up to their *en-suite* for a wank and found this book thingy hidden by the toilet – *Sensate Focus: How to pleasure your partner*. It said you had to do all this touching and feeling but only where you *didn't* want to touch. It said you had to stand naked in front of a mirror with your partner just staring at each other. The idea was that you didn't actually have sex and not having it made you want it! For a bloke-man like myself, it sounded like a load of cobblers.

But I have to admit that that is just what I did on the next pull. She's great and she's even stopped talking in sentences in bed now. What's more, with my new-found confidence I've been able to organise a piss-up in the new brewery where I work.'

Psychological issues

This man is a self-defined 'bloke-man' who, at the beginning of the scenario is suffering an all too common problem of the 21st century male – redundancy, in more ways than one. He has lost his job, his partner and his self-esteem (if not identity) due to impotence.

His medication for his high blood pressure is possibly affecting his sexual performance too. He was prescribed this in an all too brief consultation and yet when he gets the chance to discuss the 'other department' he is too embarrassed in front of the attractive nurse.

The internet provides him with his first port of call, pornographic images. Having failed to enhance his performance, he returns to the online facility of the NHS. Highly informative (and with the necessary privacy) he realises his medication could be a factor and he reads about sexual counselling. But his sense of masculinity is threatened at the thought of getting help and he imagines a scenario with an older woman talking to him.

He tries banter with a male relative. He tries one of the latest men's magazines, which serves to give him back a group identity (of some aggression) as a male struggling to satisfy women who talk in sentences in bed.

An interesting (and entertaining) article about men's magazines is *Disgrace under Pressure* by Andrew O'Hagan (*see* Further reading).

By chance he reads the book advising 'sensate focus' as a strategy to enhance sexual performance. He is bemused by the paradoxical content but discovers it works and by the end of the scenario he is happily having sex with a new girlfriend.

The word 'willy', as a generic term, has a comic connotation. Some men name their 'willies'. What do you make of the psychology of this? Is it evidence that men have a part of themselves that acts separately, if not uncontrollably, like a small animal?

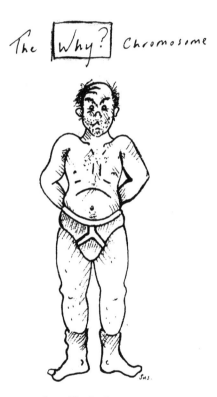

The Why? chromosome.

Personal and professional development

1 The use of humour (needing a microscope to find a penis), whilst intending to break the ice in a difficult consultation, is probably one of the greatest arts in the science of medicine! Sadly, the anecdote from a colleague contributed to this patient not seeking help at his surgery. Reflect on your use of humour in sexual consultations.

2 If you are a man, think about your attitudes to your sexual performance. If you are a woman, reflect on times when you have tried to counsel a man (in bed?) whose identity is threatened by what he perceives to be poor sexual performance. As a woman, have you felt the urge to 'perform', to fake orgasmic ecstasy while feeling deprived of intimacy?

3 The practice nurse intuitively guesses that the patient is worried about impotence but her question embarrasses him. What could have been done differently?

4 Design a health campaign for men's health, focusing on fears about sexuality.

5 Some parts of the internet and the media contribute aggressive images about sexuality. Is there a role for healthcare professionals to neutralise this effect in some way? We may have lost sight of the fact that sexual intercourse was originally designed for the creation of children.

6 The sexism in this scenario (e.g. the putdowns about women talking instead of mewing) is an example of the wider divisiveness in society still prevalent in spite of (because of?) political correctness. Reflect on sexism in the health service.

7 The three-minute consultation with the female doctor prescribing the ACE inhibitors, which may be contributing to this man's impotence, could have been different. How?

8 Review the research on ways of bringing health education *to* men (e.g. in pubs, blood pressure check-ups in shopping centres).

9 How comfortable are you in sexual consultations?

10 How comfortable are you with your own sexuality or sexual attractiveness? Do you feel coerced into thoughts about performance and failure whether or not you are a man or a woman?

(Re-read page 17 – 'We live in a sexualised society ...'.)

Useful tip

If you are suffering from erectile dysfunction, first reassure yourself that you are not alone. Ten per cent of men aged 40–70* suffer from impotence.

---

*Source: The Impotence Association. Helpline: 0870 129 0100. Website: www.informED. org.uk

Z is for Zest (for life)

'I'm in my own room in the hospice and I've just enjoyed a bowl of home-made soup. I can see trees, roses in bloom, soft-green lawns, squirrels and birds. I have never been so well treated in all my 71 years. I'm in my last few weeks of life and I am having the time of my life. The company is fantastic and that's staff, the patients and the volunteers who bring round hot drinks. One of them even plays the piano in the day room, which makes a change from the buzz from the tropical fish tank. My only worry is that I don't want to die in bed. I want to die in reception.

I used to be a lorry driver. I was on a north–south run carrying wagon loads of whisky. It was stupid of me, but I boasted one night about the cargo. I was followed down the motorway from the service station and beaten up with a crowbar. Left for dead on the hard shoulder, my life was saved by an off-duty ambulance man who got me into hospital. Compensation for the loss of my job came to £250 000 and I was warned that the blood clot left in my brain could kill me at anytime. So I spent the money on the 'good life' in a matter of years and ended up living in a caravan in Scarborough, until I met my third wife. She was the one that brought me to God (and the Open University). As far as we know, the clot's still settled comfortably somewhere in my head. But the cancer in my lungs has spread.

I'm reading the *Bible*, especially Matthew Chapter 4 verses i–xi. It's all about Christ being tempted by the devil in the wilderness. He is offered total security, approval and power if he will just subjugate himself to the devil. It made me think of how distorted these needs have become in our world. Yes, we need the security of a roof over our heads. Yes, we need friends to encourage us and approve (some of) our actions. Yes, we need strength or power, but not over others. We do not need securities, fame, domination and celebrities.

I know how to change the world . . . .

- Beckham and Posh would walk out on to a football stadium and announce that they are leaving the limelight.
- The editors of all the tabloids would agree to change their columns by a millimetre a day.

- The Royal family would appear on that balcony at Buckingham Palace and announce their disappearance from public life.

It's not the morphine talking. These may be my dreams but they are not hallucinations.

A nurse has just come in to sit with me for a while.

"My bags are packed and ready to go", I joke.
"I'm glad you're ready, Russ, because your wife's just rung to say she's sorting your party out."
"In reception?"
"Of course. We will sort everything out for you so that when the time is right, you can move down the corridor."
"Thank you. And don't forget, the only words I want in that Book of Remembrance are 'thank you'."

I was talking to the chaplain yesterday. She's had an interesting life. She once nearly died on an operating table and had a near-death experience of going down this tunnel towards the light. She said that she didn't really want to come back to earth but it was made clear to her that she had a job to do. We can only imagine what the next life will be like but I think I know. Time and space will no longer constrict us and, since with God nothing is ever lost, we will be able to walk down the streets of ancient Rome. We will see everything and everyone clearly. It will be beautiful.'

> *"Say 'yes' to today; say 'yes' to tomorrow; say 'yes' to eternity."*

Psychological issues

The quality of hospice care (private room with a view, home-made soup, excellent staff) is celebrated in this scenario. Russ is able to choose where he wants to die as well. Flexible care and liaison with his wife are ensuring the best end to his life.

He has time to reflect on his life. He has individual support from both a member of the nursing staff and the chaplain. It appears that he is being given all the time he needs to prepare himself for his final journey. He is seemingly unafraid, if not looking forward to life after death.

There is some poignancy too, in that he implies that it has taken 71 years for him to reach such a situation of care and joy. It would seem that he has had something of a chequered career and perceives the gift of his third wife, the conversion to Christianity and a degree with the Open University as turning points.

His suggestions of what life will be like after death imply a zest-for-eternal-life. We cannot know for sure what is going on in the minds of people who report near-death experiences. The controversy about biological versus meta-physical interpretations continues.

Although the care is felt to be very individualised, there is still the reference to the 'day room' and the surprise that one of the volunteers 'even' plays the piano for the patients who are usually listening to the buzz from the tropical fish tank.

Personal and professional development

1 Reflect on your experiences of caring for the dying, either in the community, hospitals or hospices.
2 Think of the different relationships experienced by Russ with:

- his wife
- the nurse
- the chaplain
- the volunteer.

In what ways are volunteers easier for patients to relate to than close relatives?
3 What do you make of Russ's ideas to change the world?
4 Can any clinician ever conclude, without doubt, whether a patient's thoughts are dreams or hallucinations?
5 How confident are you talking about death, dying, the possibility of an after-life and different religious faiths?
6 This agreement to die in reception is a true account. How far is it realistic to 'allow' patients free choice about their place of death?
7 The nurse comes in to 'sit for a while'. How comfortable are you about 'staying with' a patient (in any situation) and doing or being seen to do very little?
8 What roles do you think chaplains (and other religious workers) play in healthcare delivery today?
9 Do you believe in a life after death?
10 What do you make of near-death experiences?

Appendix 1

In choosing the entries for the A–Z of this book, inevitably many losses had to be excluded. **Lack** of something, for example being born without one of the five senses, has not been included either. The psychology of 'lack' is subtly different from that of 'loss'. Is it a duller or more muted grieving perhaps?

Here is a supplementary list (of loss and lack) which, though equally incomplete, is offered as a starting point for further thought. I have started with anger to counterbalance **Anxiety** as a key emotion in illness. I have distinguished losses in bold and lacks in plain print.

A: Anger   It is often suggested that anger stems from frustration. Equally, we can say that underlying the bravado of displays of aggression, there is a lurking fear. And what greater fear is there than loss of health (loss of well-being) and going into hospital?

B: Blood/Brother/Belief/Belonging(s)   The sight of blood, one's own or anybody else's is a graphic reminder of our mortality. To lose a sibling, however much we may be rivals, may be too close for comfort to say the least. To lose belief, whether in ourselves or in life itself, is an intangible but powerful loss. And the sense of belonging (to family, in particular) is weakened in our society, which may explain why the grasp for belongings is so tempting to fill that void.

C: Control/Child The sense of control over our bodies is donated to the medical profession the moment we cross the portals of surgeries and hospital. To lose a child through death is the highest scoring stressor. When our children grow up and leave home, we have to 'let go'.

D: Dignity   The lack of dignity of many of the world's poorest peoples is offered as an image, to contrast with the pretty pictures on the glossy brochures for private healthcare in the West.

E: Energy   The lack of the basic physiological necessities of life, e.g. water and food, is another image to add to the one above.

Some statistics to remind us of world injustice:

- 42 million people have the HIV virus
- 40 million people are starving in Africa

- 30% of women experience domestic violence
- 40% of all UK women earn £100 a week or less
- 15 million people in the UK have personal debts in excess of £5000
- there are 34 million Cambodians and 34 million landmines in Cambodia
- since 1997, in the UK, the top 10% are 3% worse off and the bottom 10% are 15% better off
- the total national household debt in the UK has reached one trillion pounds in the year 2004
- 3 billion people worldwide cook with dung, causing smoke-related diseases leading to one life being lost every 20 seconds.

[Source: the media/2004.]

F: Fertility/Fertility   To lose or lack fertility goes against our basic life force to reproduce ourselves. The helplessness that hurts so many couples in this position has led to babies being 'imported' from poorer countries to fulfil this need. To what extent could this be construed as an abuse of power in the global marketplace? (*See* Further reading for an article in *Pulse* on the role of CAM in infertility treatment.)

G: 'God'/'God'   To lose belief in 'God' (whatever our conceptualisation of this word is) and to lack belief in a wider vision for the human condition is, perhaps, the biggest danger facing the world as it moves completely into the marketplace. We used to have distinctions between the sacred and the profane; there used to be a marketplace as a separate thing, now there is a sense in which we are all just commodities in a global v/pillage.

H: Hair   Chemotherapy? Alopecia? Thinning hair with old age? If hair is our crowning glory, then losing it is as sharp a reminder as anything of our mortality.

I: Image   We are living in an image-conscious sexualised society (*see* page 17). The fact is that our bodies do change with the passage of time and there is no gym regime or moisturiser (with or without vegetable extracts) that can stop this process. Why don't we start seeing ourselves and others as creatures? We can limit the power of the media moguls.

J: Judgement   The loss of the sense of judgement can play a profound part in the suffering of the mind, particularly for people with depression. While the darkness may absorb them, a pinprick of light may also remind them of what they are losing or have lost; and yet, re-entry to the 'kingdom of the well' is barred, for what may only be a temporary period, but for what may seem like an eternity.

K: Kitten (and other pets)   Adults may be embarrassed to speak of their grief over the loss of an animal. We can learn from children, who may cry over a budgie, a tortoise or a goldfish. An interesting game to play is to recall the name of your first pet and then combine that with your mother's maiden name. Conjure yourself a new identity.

L: Limb/Limb   To lose a limb is not just to lose part of yourself but your identity. To lack a limb from birth is to be born into a world of belonging to a permanent category – the disabled. To suffer from a phantom limb means that you need to read Ramachandran on phantom limbs (*see* Further reading).

M: Men/Men   The menopause is the men-are-gone. Or is it? Women can feel a loss of confidence when their hormones start to fluctuate in middle age. You might like to look at the EBM for and against HRT.

N: Nurture   In spite of the hard work by parents in rearing their children, it is not uncommon for many people to spend their lives feeling as if they had insufficient nurture.

O: Organisation   The lack of an organised life or lifestyle can be a contributory factor to the loss of well-being. For example, accidents in the home are more likely to occur if there is physical or psychological chaos.

P: Parent/Parent   To lose a mum or a dad goes against our expectations and beliefs; we tend to believe that our parents our immortal. No matter at what age this loss occurs, we owe it to ourselves and one another to grieve as long and hard or as slow and steady as is necessary. In this 'fast-forward' world, which favours the quantification of virtually everything, we read of times it takes to recover, for example two years from a divorce (or five years if it was a difficult one). Think of the difference between divorce and loss of a partner or parent through death.

To lack a parent (or a steady carer from birth to age 18) is so common now as to be virtually the norm. What do you think will happen in the future to the generations who have experienced this start in life?

Q: Quality of life   Having a rat-race lifestyle in which quantity takes precedence over quality cannot but leave a sense of dissatisfaction, for no matter how many status symbols are purchased, there is always another designer label around the next corner waiting to fill its unenviable role (of failing to fill the happiness gap).

R: Respect   Although we have imported the American slogan of 'zero toler-ance', there remains a deep lack of respect, particularly for marginalised people in our society, our world. The schism of so many -isms remains – ageism (*see* scenarios J and X in particular), sexism, racism, etc. There is also the increasing threat to people who work for the health service from frustrated, angry patients and relatives whose expectations about care and instant access to help have been manipulated by many factors.

S: Sex/Sex   The loss or lack of a 'sex life' can be felt to be high on the agenda in British society today. Why? We are living in a sexualised society (*see* page 17) which bombards us with images of sleek tanned couples, their smiling dentition implying that they are enjoying the ultimate in sexual ecstasy. If we see these pictures in advertisements, possibly on a rainy day when we feel unattractive and inadequate, they may serve to undermine us further. They may make us question the levels of pleasure we experience with our 'partners' and drive us into the wasteland of a culture of envy.

T: Touch/Touch   The loss or lack of having somebody whom you can trust to give you hugs and cuddles (perhaps without a sexual agenda) is a denial of a large part of our humanity. 'Therapeutic touch' is used as a phrase in clinical circles to demonstrate the care we need to take with boundaries when touching our patients. How many elderly people, living alone, are denied this reminder of their continuing existence?

U: Understanding   However much science commands our respect, it must be remembered that it is merely a human god. We do not understand the mysteries of life, of birth, of death, of sickness, of healing. Instead of claiming an erroneous 'understanding', perhaps we could try a little 'overfalling'. We could do worse than to fall over, metaphorically speaking, and regain some awe and wonder that we exist at all.

V: Vision/Vision/Values   The loss of sight or lack of sight from birth is a major disability. While there are many technological and emotional supports available, partially sighted or blind people remain vulnerable. A lack of humanitarian values in any individual cannot but affect the whole of humanity because we are all interconnected.

W: Willpower (to change)   If we ascribe to the branch of psychology known as 'evolutionary psychology' then we may also be accepting that it is part of our natural development to evolve as individuals throughout life. To what extent can we change ourselves? There is an increasing volume of books available in the marketplace under the category of 'self-help'. Too many of these would seem to offer quick 'n' easy answers to the human condition. Perhaps we vary, both as individuals and depending on the time and place in which we find ourselves, in the degree to which we can access our willpower. For example, changing dietary habits, giving up smoking and breaking addictions, all require a steady and consistent commitment.

X: Excitement is missing in many lives, or there can be a sense created by the media that everyone else is having a better time with everyone else. This assumption or anxiety may be a contributory factor in the ingestion of 'designer' drugs.

Y: Why can't we appreciate the things we do have? Living in the richest part of our planet, it is arguable that we should not complain about lack or loss. Everything here is luxury if compared with the poor of the Third World, for example.

Z: zzzzzz   Loss, or lack of sleep, does not add to well-being (*see* Further reading – *Counting Sheep* by Paul Martin).

Appendix 2

Here is an A–Z of suggestions for helping yourself and/or others to 'come to terms with' loss.

A: Ask for help (not necessarily professional).

B: Be kind to yourself.

C: Count the good things you do have.

D: Do something (legal!) that you have never done before.

E: Energy. Don't be surprised if you feel sapped. Grief can be hard work.

F: Friends are invaluable. Enjoy old ones and make new ones. This may be difficult if your confidence is reduced or if you are shy; your courage could be rewarded in the most unexpected ways.

G: Go for a walk in the fresh air. The four walls can be the worst place if you feel low.

H: Hold on … change is stressful … try and keep some things constant in your life.

I: If you are helping somebody else, don't be afraid just to be there without saying very much.

J: Join a club/group/society of like-minded people, if you are a club-joining sort of person. Or go online and see if there is a (safe) group/interest you could link with.

K: Keep going …………… and going …………… and going.

L: Love yourself. It is a cliché. You could start with *liking* yourself. Why not write a list or draw pictures of all the good things about yourself. 'Love' has become a word whose weight and flight have become inadequate to the task of conveying meaning, partly due to overuse and partly because its connotation is nearly always romantic or sexual. If you have been hurt by the loss or lack of love, then it may be easier to begin by neutralising the emotion, 'love', and to think about liking instead.

M: Mantras (or keeping up a positive inner dialogue with yourself) can be helpful. Saying: 'Yes I am getting better', 'Things will get easier', 'I am doing the best I can' and so on, are certainly more conducive to progress than (inadvertently) dwelling on the negative.

N: Sometimes you may need to say 'No' even if it does feel uncomfortable. Perhaps you are trying to rebuild a social life in a new job and a new town. You may fear that if you say 'No' to an invitation, you will not be asked again.

O: Open up to somebody you trust

P: Pace yourself. Take one step at a time. If it helps, you might like to record how far you have come by drawing a map, where the point-of-the-loss-incident is shaded black and the point where you are now is a paler shade of grey. Then you can visualise the route you are trying to take to the restoration of the full colour of the spectrum of life.

Q: The questions. *How can we rebuild a sense of community?* This sense is probably the sociological antidote to many of the losses experienced by people in the last 50 or so years. It could be the solution to the loneliness in our society; the loneliness which may be the primary driver pushing people into impoverished one-on-one relationships, which then break down because of the inordinately stressful demands placed on them to satisfy both partners. An answer to loneliness is solitude. There is a community of texters via the advent of mobile phones but can a 'cybernautical' relationship ever replace face-to-face encounters? 'I text therefore I am' is not necessarily the only way forward. *How can we reduce the dehumanising effects of what we might call the 'karmic plaque' of capitalism in the last 500 years?*

R: Resources? You may have more inner resources than you imagine. You may need to dig deep.

S: Soak in a warm bath or take a refreshing shower.

T: Treat yourself. Why not have some chocolate now or a healthy banana? Even if you are feeling pressurised to diet, a small treat regularly can lift your spirits.

U: Unhappiness cannot last forever! An advantage of going through the arduous process of grief is that you may be able to appreciate simpler pleasures. And having suffered, you are likely to be more sympathetic to other people in a similar situation and also more appreciative of what you do have.

V: Violent feelings are not unusual. Violent desires to replace what you have lost may entrap you for years (for example, there is the strong tendency to rebound into an inappropriate relationship shortly after the ending of a close relationship). Everybody is unique in the way they respond to these forces. In the early stages of grief, you may find that not only are you struggling with the acute suffering but also with the attempt to find some strategies to survive the emotional turmoil. Sadness (the 'softer' emotion) and anger (the 'harder' emotion) may lead to bitterness if you are very unlucky. Bitterness can be very hard to melt down and a vicious circle of cynicism and even despair can blacken your chances of being able to trust or to hope in the life-enhancing properties of friendship. When Byron spoke of friendship being love but without love's wings, he was offering us an insight into the difference between the relative ease of friendships compared with the passionate, but more risky experience of intimate relationships. On a cautionary note, it is worth remembering that while there may be a lot of friendliness in our world, real friendship is rare. 'Hold a true friend with both hands' is a Nigerian proverb.

W: Why me? Perhaps everybody asks this at some point. There are no easy answers. It can help to remind yourself that you are not alone. We are all in it together, this life, this journey; or perhaps a better term is 'ramble' since we are all vulnerable to the scratches of the brambles along the way.

X: Xmas can be a difficult time. You may need to plan in advance.

Y: You matter whether it feels like it or not; reminding somebody else that they matter too, when struggling with grief, even in the smallest possible way, is a big help in the healing process.

Z: Zzzzzzzzzzz and rest are necessary. Grief is hard work.

Appendix 3

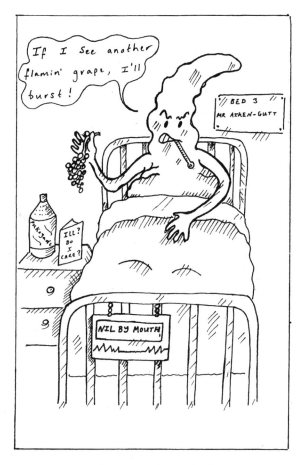

The appendix in bed 3.

Further reading

Introduction to psychology

Gross R (2001) *Psychology. The Science of Mind and Behaviour* (4e). Hodder & Stoughton, London.

Selwyn M (1994) *The Awakening Year: an exploration in Gestalt psychotherapy*. Hodder Headline, London.

Advanced psychology

Neimeyer R (2001) *Meaning Reconstruction and the Experience of Loss*. American Psychological Association, Washington DC.

Books and articles on death, dying, grief, bereavement and suicide

Boss P (1999) *Ambiguous Loss*. Harvard University Press, Cambridge, MA.

Callanan M and Kelley P (1992) *Final Gifts: understanding and helping the dying*. Hodder & Stoughton, London.

Dickenson D, Johnson M and Samson Katz J (2000) *Death, Dying and Bereavement* (2e). Open University, Buckingham.

Horn S (1989) *Coping with Bereavement*. Thorsons Publishing Group, London.

Ironside V (1996) *'You'll Get Over It'*. Penguin, London.

Lake T (1984) *Living with Grief*. Sheldon Press, London.

Murray Parkes C (1996) *Bereavement: studies of grief in adult life*. Penguin, London.

Neuberger J (2004) *Caring for Dying People of Different Faiths*. Radcliffe Medical Press, Oxford.

Neuberger J (2004) *Dying Well: a guide to enabling a good death* (2e). Radcliffe Medical Press, Oxford.

Simmons M (ed.) (2000) *Getting a Life: older people talking*. Peter Owen Publishers/ Help the Aged, London.

Ward B (1993) *Healing Grief*. Vermilion, London.

Wilkinson (1999) Notes left behind (the language of suicide). *The New Yorker.* 15 February.

Worden W (1983) *Grief Counselling and Grief Therapy.* Tavistock, London.

Other books and articles relevant to loss

Anonymous author/ex-junior hospital doctor (2001) Why am I crying? *BMJ.* **323:** 1010.

Bruce EJ and Schultz CL (2001) *Nonfinite Loss and Grief: a psychoeducational approach.* Jessica Kingsley Publishers, London.

Butler G and Hope T (1995) *Manage your Mind.* Oxford University Press, Oxford.

Coulson C and Jenkins J (2004) The role of complementary and alternative medicine (in the treatment of infertility). *Pulse.* **64(6):** 56–9.

Dorland WAN (1923) *The American Illustrated Medical Dictionary* (12e). WB Saunders. Philadelphia and London.

Edwards N, Kornacki MJ and Silversin J (2002) Unhappy doctors: what are the causes and what can be done? *BMJ.* **324:** 835–8.

Finegan W (2004) *Trust Me, I'm a ~~Doctor~~ Cancer Patient.* Radcliffe Medical Press, Oxford.

Groopman J (2002) Dying words: how should doctors deliver bad news? *The New Yorker,* 28 October.

Groopman J (2004) The grief industry: how much does crisis counselling help or hurt? *The New Yorker,* 22 January.

Hodgkinson T (2004) Branded for life: a review of *Willing Slaves: how the overwork culture is ruling our lives. Guardian.* 3 July.

Jackson J (2001) *Truth, Trust and Medicine.* Routledge, London.

Jacobsen FW, Kindlen M and Shoemark A (1997) *Living Through Loss: manual for those working with issues of terminal illness and bereavement.* Jessica Kingsley Publishers, London.

James O (2002) *They Fuck You Up: how to survive family life.* Bloomsbury, London.

Kovel J (1992) *A Complete Guide to Therapy.* Penguin, London.

Kuhse H and Singer P (eds) (1999) *Bioethics, an Anthology.* Blackwell, Oxford.

Levenkron S (2001) *Anatomy of Anorexia.* WW Norton, New York.

Mallon B (1998) *Helping Children to Manage Loss: positive strategies for renewal and growth.* Jessica Kingsley Publishers, London.

Martin P (2002) *Counting Sheep.* Flamingo/Harper Collins, London.

Murray CJL and Lopez AD (eds) (1996) *The Global Burden of Disease: a comprehensive assessment of mortality and disability from diseases, injuries and risk factors in 1990 and projected to 2020.* Harvard School of Public Health on behalf of the WHO and the World Bank (Global Burden of Disease and Injury Series Vol I), Cambridge, MA.

Newton L (1981) In defense of the traditional nurse. *Nursing Outlook.* **29(6):** 348–54.

O'Neill O (2002) *A Question of Trust: the BBC Reith Lectures.* Cambridge University Press, Cambridge.

Ramachandran V (1999) *Phantoms in the Brain.* Fourth Estate/Harper Collins, London.

Rungapadiachy D (1999) *Interpersonal Communication and Psychology for Healthcare Professionals*. Butterworth-Heinemann, Oxford.

Sacks O (1985) *The Man Who Mistook His Wife for a Hat*. Picador, London.

Slater L (2004) Into the Cuckoo's Nest. *Guardian Weekend*, 31 January.

Smail D (1987) *Taking Care*. Dent, London.

Smail D (1993) *The Origins of Unhappiness*. Harper Collins, London.

Treasure J (1997) *Anorexia Nervosa*. Psychology Press Ltd, Hove.

Widgery D (1988) *The National Health Service: a radical perspective*. The Hogarth Press, London.

Wolpert L (1999) *Malignant Sadness: the anatomy of depression*. Faber & Faber, London.

Zimbardo PG (1990) *Shyness: what it is and what to do about it*. Addison-Wesley Publishing Company, Reading, MA.

Wider literature (with the common theme of loss or survival of same)

Alighieri D (1948) *The Divine Comedy*. Pantheon Books, New York. First published 1301.

Astley N (ed.) (2002) *Staying Alive*. Bloodaxe Books, Newcastle upon Tyne.

Bauman, Z (2003) *Liquid Love*. Polity, Cambridge.

de Botton A (1998) *How Proust Can Change your Life*. Pan/MacMillan, London.

de Botton A (2000) *The Consolations of Philosophy*. Penguin, London.

de Botton A (2004) *Status Anxiety*. Hamish Hamilton, London.

Bunting M (2004) *Willing Slaves: how the overwork culture is ruling our lives*. Harper Collins, London.

Cawley AC (ed.) (1993) *Everyman and medieval miracle plays*. Dent, London.

Cusk R (1995) *The Temporary*. Picador, London.

Daneman M (1993) *The Favourite*. Faber & Faber, London.

Forbes P (ed.) 2003) *We Have Come Through*. Bloodaxe Books, Newcastle upon Tyne.

Hutton W (1995) *The State We're In*. Vintage, London.

Larkin P (1988) *Collected Poems*. Faber & Faber, London.

Lewis J (1941) *The Wife of Martin Guerre*. Penguin, London.

Lodge D (1995)*Therapy: a novel*. Secker & Warburg Ltd, London.

McEwan I (1987) *The Child in Time*. Vintage, London.

Milton J (2004) *Paradise Lost*. (eds) J Goldberg and S Orgel. Oxford University Press, Oxford.

O'Farrell (2001) *After You'd Gone*. Headline, London.

O'Hagan A (2004) Disgrace under pressure. *London Review of Books*, 3 June.

Radcliffe T (2001) *I Call You Friends*. Continuum, London/New York.

Rhys J (1972) *Tigers are Better-Looking* (recommended story: Outside the Machine). Penguin, London.

Rubens B (1991) *A Solitary Grief*. Abacus, London.
Rubens B (2002) *Nine Lives*. Abacus, London.
Rubens B (1997) *The Waiting Game*. Abacus, London.
Sayer P (1988) *The Comforts of Madness*. Sceptre, London.
Shields C (2003) *Unless*. Harper Collins, London.
Updike J (1968) *Couples*. Penguin, London.

Health is defined in the WHO
Constitution as 'a state of complete
physical, mental and social well-being
and not merely the absence of disease
or infirmity'.

Index

3